Let's Talk

Let's Talk

Navigating Communication Services and Supports for Your Young Child with Autism

by

Rhea Paul, Ph.D., CCC-SLP
Sacred Heart University
Fairfield, Connecticut

and

Donia Fahim, Ph.D.
New York University
New York, New York

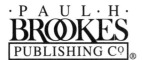

·P·A·U·L·H·
BROOKES
PUBLISHING CO.®

Baltimore • London • Sydney

2830835

MAR 31 2016

·P A U L·H·
BROOKES
PUBLISHING C°®

Paul H. Brookes Publishing Co.
Post Office Box 10624
Baltimore, Maryland 21285-0624

www.brookespublishing.com

Typeset by Scribe, Inc., Philadelphia, Pennsylvania.
Manufactured in the United States of America by
Sheridan Books, Inc., Chelsea, Michigan.

All illustrations by Maiko Suzuki.
Clip art is © istockphoto.com.
Cover image is © istockphoto/PeopleImages.

All examples in this book are composites. Any similarity to actual individuals or circumstances is
coincidental, and no implications should be inferred.

Library of Congress Cataloging-in-Publication Data

The Library of Congress has cataloged the print edition as follows:

Paul, Rhea, author.

   Let's talk: navigating communication services and supports for your young child with autism / Rhea Paul,
Ph.D., CCC-SLP, Sacred Heart University, Fairfield, Connecticut, and Donia Fahim, Ph.D., New York
University, New York, NY.
     pages   cm
   Includes bibliographical references and index.
   ISBN 978-1-59857-120-2 (paperback) — ISBN 978-1-68125-035-9 (pdf e-book)
   1. Autism in children.   2. Autistic children—Care.   3. Autistic children—Family relationships.   I. Fahim,
Donia, author.   II. Title.

RJ506.A9P38 2016

618.92'85882—dc23   2015018504

British Library Cataloguing in Publication data are available from the British Library.

2019   2018   2017   2016   2015

10   9   8   7   6   5   4   3   2   1

Contents

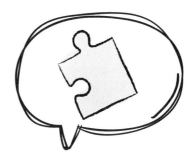

About the Authors

Rhea Paul, Ph.D., CCC-SLP, is Professor and Founding Director of the Speech-Language Pathology graduate program at Sacred Heart University in Fairfield, Connecticut; an affiliate at Haskins Laboratories; and Professor Emerita at Southern Connecticut State University. She received her bachelor's degree from Brandeis University in Waltham, Massachusetts; her master's degree in reading and learning disabilities from the Harvard Graduate School of Education in Cambridge, Massachusetts; and her doctoral degree in Communication Disorders from the University of Wisconsin–Madison. She has been a principal investigator on research projects on language disorders and autism funded by the National Institute on Deafness and Other Communication Disorders, the National Institute of Child Health and Human Development, Autism Speaks, the Meyer Memorial Trust, the Oregon Medical Foundation, and at the Yale Autism Center of Excellence.

Dr. Paul is the author of more than 90 refereed journal articles, 40 book chapters, and eight books. She received the Editor's Award from the *American Journal of Speech-Language Pathology* in 1996 and was awarded the inaugural Ritvo/Slifka Award for Innovative Clinical Research by the International Society for Autism Research in 2010. Dr. Paul has been a Fellow of the American Speech-Language Hearing-Association since 1991 and received the Honors of the Association in 2014.

Donia Fahim, Ph.D., is Senior Consultant for the ASD Nest Project at Steinhardt School of Culture, Education, and Human Development at New York University and Assistant Professor at Hunter College in New York City, where she was Program Coordinator for the Early Childhood Special Education Program from 2008 to 2013. She is also Cofounder and Executive Director of Autism Friendly Spaces and developer of the first dual language ASD Next public school program in New York City. She obtained her bachelor's, master's, and doctoral degrees from the University of London, England. She is a certified member of the Royal College of Speech and Language Therapists.

For the last 20 years, Dr. Fahim has worked as an international consultant in speech-language pathology. She served as Clinical Director and Founding Member of The Egyptian Society for Developing Skills of Special Needs Children from 1998 to 2007, focusing on work with individuals with autism spectrum disorder (ASD) and early intervention. She developed organization-specific educational curriculum, clinical procedures, and guidelines for special education for young children with special needs (e.g., Egypt: Advance Society, Learning Resource Center, Nida Center, Caritas; Saudi Arabia: Saudi Autistic Society; Nigeria: Patrick Center; Jordan: Early Years Center, Monetessori School of Amman). As a Global Master Trainer for the United Nations Children's Fund (UNICEF) in Early Childhood Development in Emergency, she has provided and consulted on speech-language pathology services throughout the world, most often in the Middle East and Africa.

Dr. Fahim has appeared on national and international radio and television in the United States, Africa, and Asia. She has been an invited speaker at many leading international conferences and events hosted by both governmental and nongovernmental organizations, such as the National Council for Motherhood and Childhood in Egypt; the United Nations Educational, Scientific and Cultural Organization Education for All (UNESCO EFA) conferences (Beirut); the Annual Autism Conference in Egypt; the World Autism Congress and Exhibition in South Africa; the Stockholm Annual Autism Conference; and the Saudi Autism awareness campaign. She was a keynote speaker at the 2014 Saudi International Occupational Therapy Conference and also received awards from the Saudi ministry of health for her contribution to parent training for families of children with ASD.

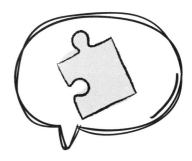

Prologue

If you're reading this book, chances are it's because you've found out that someone in your family has autism spectrum disorder (ASD) and you are feeling the need to learn as much as you can as quickly as you can about this condition and how to handle it. Our aim is to try to give you the information you need in a straightforward way. We've tried to describe ASD, define the various terms clinicians use, show how ASD affects a child's development and learning, relay what we know about treating its symptoms, and provide guidance on how to talk to the professionals you will meet as you construct the best program for your child. We've also tried to talk about how it feels to families, because the needs of other family members sometimes get overshadowed with all of the attention on the child who has been diagnosed with ASD.

The best advice we can give families just starting this journey is to take a breath! We know it feels as if you have to do everything now perfectly or your child's chances for success will be diminished. You're probably worrying that if you lose a day or a week of programming, then you'll limit your child's chances for success. Yet, this is not a sprint; it's a marathon. Pace yourself. Do what you can, but don't worry about what you can't do. Yes, early intervention is certainly important, but if it starts in a month instead of this week, your child will still derive significant benefit. The most important thing for your child with ASD is exactly the same thing that's most important for any other child—to have strong and loving parents with the mental and physical health to provide a safe and stable home. So, taking care of your own physical and mental health is just as important as what you put in place for your child. In the course of this book, we'll provide information to help you organize the programming your child will need to develop and learn. You have time—it really doesn't all have to happen today. In the meantime, you should think just as hard about what to do for yourself, your partner, and your other children to make sure everyone can blossom in the environment you create for your child with ASD. We sincerely hope that this book will play some small part in helping you to fashion a place where your child and your family can thrive.

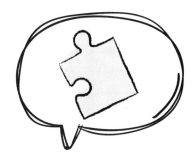

Acknowledgments

We want to express our appreciation to Amanda Rizzo for her editorial assistance in preparing this manuscript. We also thank everyone at Paul H. Brookes Publishing Co. for their patience and support throughout the process. To our colleagues and students at the Yale Child Study Center, Hunter College, New York University, and Sacred Heart University, we are grateful for all you have taught us and all you have goaded us to learn.

*To all the devoted and courageous families who,
through raising children with ASD, have taught us so much*

What Is Autism Spectrum Disorder, and How Is It Diagnosed?

Jason was Mariana and Joe's second child. Their first child, Molly, seemed to do everything early. She walked and talked just after her first birthday, and at 3 years old, when Jason was born, she was an adorable little chatterbox with a lot of friends at preschool and in the neighborhood. Jason was a more challenging infant than Molly had been from day one. He didn't sleep through the night for what seemed to his parents like forever, and he was fussy and more upset by changes in the daily routine. But he reached all his motor milestones—turning over, sitting up, and walking—at about the same time as Molly. Mariana couldn't help feeling concerned, though, when Jason was 18 months old and hadn't started talking. Everyone told her it was just because he was a boy and they talked later than girls. It wasn't just the talking, though. He didn't seem to hear when she spoke to him, he wasn't able to follow simple directions as Molly had at his age, and he didn't answer when Mariana called his name. At Jason's 18-month checkup, the pediatrician suggested he have his hearing tested.

Mariana felt relieved; the doctor agreed everything was not as it should be, and if Jason were deaf, then there were things to do about that. The audiologist who tested Jason explained that he did not have a hearing loss, however. On hearing this, Mariana was shocked to find herself in tears. What was wrong with her? She should be happy that he wasn't deaf. Yet if he could hear, then why wasn't he learning to talk? Why didn't he listen or understand when others spoke? Now other behaviors she'd been worrying about—things she'd pushed to the back of her mind or chalked up to his being a boy—came crowding into her head. He seemed to prefer to play on his own and didn't seek out other children; sometimes he actively avoided them when they were around. And he was so rigid, such as the time she had made cupcakes with pink icing for Molly's birthday and he had a temper tantrum and threw his cupcake on the floor because she had always made cupcakes with white icing. What could be wrong? What could she do about it?

Does this scenario (or parts of it) sound familiar? If you've been through similar experiences, you've probably guessed that Jason was eventually diagnosed with autism spectrum disorder (ASD). It may even seem obvious to you now, but Jason's behavior could be mystifying for parents who have little prior experience with ASD. He seems to be developing well in some ways, but he lags far behind his peers in other ways. He can see and hear, but he uses his senses differently than other children. And most crucially, he isn't attracted to people. This is the central problem and the defining feature of autism—a reduced drive to interact with others; to share enjoyment, thoughts, and feelings with others; and to be like others. There are other symptoms, too, as we'll see, but this deficit in social-communication is at the core of autism. Let's look at some of the definitions of ASD and learn how professionals decide that a child has this disorder.

MY CHILD WAS DIAGNOSED WITH ASD—WHAT DOES THAT MEAN?

Definitions of autism have gone through a lot of changes since the disorder was first recognized by the psychiatrist Leo Kanner in 1943. Kanner identified two primary symptoms of autism. A profound difficulty in relating to others was the first symptom. Kanner noted that this core deficit in social ability was accompanied by a range of problems in using language as a means of social interaction as well as in using other nonverbal forms of communication from very early in life. An excessive insistence on sameness and repetitive activities—such as rocking, spinning, or lining things up—or interests, which led to severe limitations in the variety of spontaneous activities in which the child would participate, was the second core symptom noted in Kanner's original description of the 11 children he identified as having this "new" syndrome.

Of course, autism existed before Kanner discovered it. Uta Frith, a prominent autism expert, wrote that Victor, a child found living alone in the woods in France around 1800, was likely to have had autism. Victor was taken in by a prominent physician who tried to educate him (with very limited success) and was the subject of several books and movies, including Francois Truffaut's (1970) "The Wild Child." Harlan Lane, author of *The Wild Boy of Aveyron,* a book about Victor, suggested that many children found wandering alone and thought to be raised by animals were probably abandoned by their families as a result of their severe autism, for which there were no effective treatments.

Although there have been children with autism as long as there have been children, Kanner's contribution recognized commonalities among symptoms seen in children at different levels of function, observing that they all showed the same general problems in social interaction, communication, and rigid repetitiveness, regardless of whether they could speak. Moreover, he was able to discern that their deficits in social interaction and rigidity were above and beyond those seen in children with intellectual disabilities (ID) alone and couldn't be entirely accounted for by low cognitive skills because even children with severe cognitive impairments were drawn to others and communicated through gesture, sound, and gaze, if not through words.

Although technical definitions have changed over the years, the two core problems Kanner identified have remained at the heart of diagnostic classifications of autism. The *Diagnostic and Statistical Manual of Mental Disorders, Fifth Edition* (*DSM-5*; American Psychiatric Association, 2013) focuses more directly than previous versions on these two primary symptoms. Box 1.1 presents the *DSM-5* definition, which contains the diagnostic criteria currently used by medical professionals.

 ## The *DSM-5* (American Psychiatric Association, 2013) Diagnostic Criteria for Autism Spectrum Disorder

A. Persistent deficits in social communication and social interaction across multiple contexts, as manifested by the following, currently or by history (examples are illustrative, not exhaustive; all three symptoms must be present):

   1. Deficits in social-emotional reciprocity, ranging, for example, from abnormal social approach and failure of normal back-and-forth conversation; to reduced sharing of interests, emotions, or affect; to failure to initiate or respond to social interactions.

   2. Deficits in nonverbal communicative behaviors used for social interaction, ranging, for example, from poorly integrated verbal and nonverbal communication; to abnormalities in eye contact and body language or deficits in understanding and use of gestures; to a total lack of facial expressions and nonverbal communication.

   3. Deficits in developing, maintaining, and understanding relationships, ranging, for example, from difficulties adjusting behavior to suit various social contexts; to difficulties in sharing imaginative play or in making friends; to absence of interest in peers.

B. Restricted, repetitive patterns of behavior, interests, or activities, as manifested by at least two of the following, currently or by history (examples are illustrative, not exhaustive; two of the four symptoms must be present):

(continued)

BOX 1.1 *(continued)*

   1. Stereotyped or repetitive motor movements, use of objects, or speech (e.g., simple motor stereotypies, lining up toys or flipping objects, echolalia, idiosyncratic phrases).

   2. Insistence on sameness, inflexible adherence to routines, or ritualized patterns or verbal nonverbal behavior (e.g., extreme distress at small changes, difficulties with transitions, rigid thinking patterns, greeting rituals, need to take same route or eat the same food every day).

   3. Highly restricted, fixated interests that are abnormal in intensity or focus (e.g., strong attachment to or preoccupation with unusual objects, excessively circumscribed or perseverative interest).

   4. Hyper- or hypo-reactivity to sensory input or unusual interests in sensory aspects of the environment (e.g., apparent indifference to pain/temperature, adverse response to specific sounds or textures, excessive smelling or touching of objects, visual fascination with lights or movement).

C. Symptoms must be present in the early developmental period (but may not become fully manifest until social demands exceed limited capacities, or may be masked by learned strategies in later life).

D. Symptoms cause clinically significant impairment in social, occupational, or other important areas of current functioning.

E. These disturbances are not better explained by intellectual disability (intellectual developmental disorder) or global developmental delay. Intellectual disability and autism spectrum disorder frequently co-occur; to make comorbid diagnoses of autism spectrum disorder and intellectual disability, social communication should be below that expected for general developmental level.

The *DSM-5* (American Psychiatric Association, 2013) is the volume written by committees of the American Psychiatric Association, the main professional group for psychiatrists in the United States. The manual is used by psychiatrists, psychologists, and others who deal with mental health to define the characteristics of mental illnesses, state the diagnostic criteria that research suggests are most valid for each, and provide guidance to practitioners in making diagnoses. The manual is updated as new research is gathered that helps to refine diagnostic criteria and as society changes its views. For example, there was a category called *mental retardation* in the *DSM-IV* that was used to identify people with cognitive limitations severe enough to affect their ability to learn in typical classrooms and live independently. This condition is called *intellectual disability,* however, in the *DSM-5* because societal norms changed. The term *mental retardation* was seen as negative, and advocates favored a more neutral term that carried fewer undesirable undertones and couldn't be used as an insult. *Intellectual disability* is a term that advocates find more acceptable. Similarly, homosexuality was listed as a mental disorder in earlier versions of the *DSM* but has been removed because our culture now views it as a normal variation of human behavior rather than a disease.

What Does It Mean to Say My Child Is "On the Spectrum?"

ASD is the only condition of its type described in the *DSM-5* (American Psychiatric Association, 2013; see Box 1.1). If your child is old enough to have been diagnosed a few years ago, though, you might have heard other terms being discussed. The following sections address these other terms, even though they aren't part of the *DSM-5* criteria.

Pervasive Developmental Disorder   Pervasive developmental disorder (PDD) was used to include the full autism spectrum. Because diagnostic criteria for autism were somewhat more restrictive in the *DSM-IV* (1994), PDD was used as an umbrella term to cover autism that was more strictly defined and other forms of severe developmental disorders that presented with similar symptoms. The *DSM-IV* listed several separate disorders under the umbrella of PDD, including the following.

Autism, or Autistic Disorder   Children were given a diagnosis of autism, sometimes called *classic autism,* in earlier diagnostic systems, including the *DSM-IV* (1994), if they appeared to exhibit all of the core symptoms of ASD with sufficient severity. Children with some symptoms of autism who did not meet the criteria for the full-blown syndrome were given other diagnostic labels. Autism is considered a spectrum, however, in the *DSM-5* (American Psychiatric Association, 2013) because it has a wide range of severity levels in children with a broad range of cognitive abilities, from severe impairments to high intellectual functioning. Any child showing both social-communicative deficits and restricted, repetitive

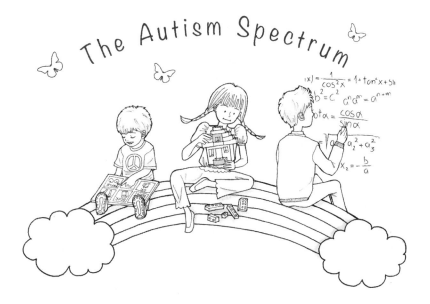

patterns of behaviors, interests, and activities—regardless of severity or level of cognitive function—is considered to have a disorder on the autism spectrum and will be diagnosed with ASD by the *DSM-5* criteria.

Pervasive Developmental Disorder—Not Otherwise Specified   In earlier diagnostic schemes, pervasive developmental disorder—not otherwise specified (PDD-NOS) was a diagnosis given to children with milder, more limited symptoms in core deficit areas or with symptoms in some areas but not all. PDD-NOS turned out to be a more common diagnosis than full-blown autism because it could be given even to children who didn't show all the required symptoms. PDD-NOS was eliminated, however, in the *DSM-5* (American Psychiatric Association, 2013). Children who show social-communication disorders without rigid, repetitive behaviors are now diagnosed with social-communication disorder, although the validity of this classification is still a matter of debate (Norbury, 2014.) If both social-communication and restricted/repetitive behaviors are present, then a diagnosis of ASD is made in the *DSM-5* scheme, regardless of the level of severity of the symptoms.

Asperger Syndrome   Asperger syndrome is another controversial diagnosis. Before the *DSM-5* (American Psychiatric Association, 2013), it was typically used for children with significant social disabilities and restricted and repetitive behaviors and interests but without any ID or language delay. These children often were not identified until they were school-age because they learned language at the usual time and their intense interests and "little professor" qualities made them appear cute or precocious rather than impaired as young children. Their social deficits became more problematic as they attempted to form peer relationships, however, and their rigidity could cause problems in school settings. These issues often triggered a referral for diagnostic assessment during the elementary or middle school years.

The syndrome was named after an Austrian doctor who in 1944 identified a group of boys who showed social disabilities similar to those Kanner described, but were intelligent and had good language skills. Because Kanner and Asperger never met or discussed their cases, it has always been unclear whether the boys Asperger identified had the same condition as Kanner's children but were simply at the high end of the spectrum, or whether their condition was really different from Kanner's autism. Asperger's work received more attention when it was translated into English in the 1990s, and a syndrome of social disability in the presence of high cognitive and language skills was named after him and included in the *DSM-IV (1994)*. Controversy continued about whether this was really different from autism. A decision was made, over strong objections from some autism experts, to drop Asperger syndrome as a separate disorder in the *DSM-5* (American Psychiatric Association, 2013) and to identify people like those described in Asperger's work as having ASD. Although many people are still unhappy about this decision, it was made because research showed there wasn't much difference in the need for support or in the long-range outcome between children who were identified as having Asperger syndrome and those with typical cognitive functioning who were given a diagnosis of high-functioning autism.

Rett Syndrome　　Rett syndrome is a rare (about 1 in 20,000; Volkmar, Reichow, Westphal, & Mandell, 2014) genetic neurological disorder that almost exclusively affects girls. It shares several features with autism, including repetitive movements, particularly of the hands, inconsolable crying, avoidance of eye contact, lack of social engagement, and failure to develop speech. It was included as a PDD in *DSM-IV (1994)*. Research has found, however, that it is caused by the mutation of a single gene, unlike autism. Rett syndrome is, unfortunately, a degenerative disorder in which children usually do not survive to adulthood. Even though it shares some symptoms with ASD, it was excluded from the *DSM-5* (American Psychiatric Association, 2013) primarily because its biological mechanisms appear to be different from those in ASD.

Childhood Disintegrative Disorder　　Childhood disintegrative disorder (CDD) was first described by Theodor Heller in 1908, 35 years before autism was recognized as a syndrome, and is sometimes called Heller's syndrome. After a period of typical development, children with CDD begin to lose skills, usually between 3 and 7 years of age. The regression can be dramatic, and the child may be aware of it and ask questions about it. Many of these children go through periods of extreme anxiety or even appear to have hallucinations; they may show hyperactivity, aggression, and lose motor skills. The outcome is usually a loss of most speech and a lifelong severe level of impairment (Volkmar et al., 2014). Thankfully, this condition is quite rare, appearing in about 1 out of 50,000 children, or 1 out of every 189 cases of autism (Hill, Zuckerman, & Fombonne, 2014). Again, the *DSM-5* (American Psychiatric Association, 2013) provides no separate category for CDD. Children who show this kind of late onset regression are given the same ASD diagnosis as any other child with the syndrome in the *DSM-5* scheme.

HOW DO PROFESSIONALS DECIDE WHETHER A CHILD HAS ASD?

After Jason's hearing test, Mariana decided she had waited long enough. She needed a better understanding of Jason's behavior, and if he needed help, then she wanted to start getting it for him. She called her pediatrician's office and talked about her concerns with the nurse, who referred her to the local birth-to-3 agency to request a developmental evaluation.

The birth-to-3 team, including an early intervention specialist, speech-language pathologist (SLP), and occupational therapist (OT), came to their home. Mariana didn't know what to expect, but whatever it was, it didn't include their bringing a huge plastic box of toys and each individual sitting and playing with Jason. The team seemed determined to frustrate him, putting treats in jars he couldn't open, activating mechanical toys without warning that startled him, and pointing to pictures in which Jason seemed uninterested. They didn't seem to try to get him to talk—although they did call his name several times to see if he would answer—or count or do any of the things children are supposed to be able to do. Mariana couldn't understand what they were after or how it would help them learn about Jason's problems.

There is no test for autism. Unlike other conditions, such as celiac disease, which can be identified by a blood test, or ID, which is diagnosed with a combination of standardized IQ and adaptive behavior testing, there is no test that tells us definitively whether autism is present. Because the symptoms of autism are based in the child's behavior and include what children do (e.g., repetitive behaviors) and what they don't do (e.g., respond to their name, use eye contact, seek out play with peers), making a diagnosis requires an extended and detailed observation of behaviors, including trying to elicit behaviors that we know don't occur in children with the syndrome.

This process can be frustrating when parents have to watch their child being asked to do exactly the things they know he or she is not good at, as well as see the examiners enable him or her to engage in some of the behaviors that are most troubling, such as spinning or peering at parts of objects. There just isn't any other way to know if a child has autism because those troublesome behaviors are the main signs of the disorder. It can't be detected by any medical test. It also can't be identified by using the kinds of cognitive problems that are part of IQ tests, such as having children imitate block designs, because many children with ASD are quite good at these skills. The only way to demonstrate that a child has ASD is to look for deficits in social interaction (e.g., looking at others, sharing enjoyment with others) and communication (e.g., talking spontaneously, following directions, asking others for things, telling others what interests them, carrying on back-and-forth conversations) and the presence of rigid and repetitive behaviors (e.g., resisting change, peering at objects, performing repetitive motor movements, displaying echoed speech). This means these behaviors sometimes need to be brought out or tolerated so they can be seen and evaluated. That's why your team will use an evaluation protocol that attempts to get a look at the behaviors most characteristic of ASD.

Behavior Observation and Parent Support

There are two ways a team gets the needed information about a child's behavior to determine whether a diagnosis of ASD is warranted. First, team members observe the child and try to create situations that will bring out the unusual behaviors that characterize the syndrome. Second, the team asks parents detailed questions about their child's behaviors—those that would be expected in typical development and those that are indicative of ASD—and about when important milestones of development, such as crawling and walking, first took place.

Neither of these methods is perfect, of course. Direct observation of behavior might miss important symptoms that the child just doesn't happen to show during a brief clinical session, or children may seem to show more severe impairments because they are upset by the change in their usual routine. Using parent report can avoid both of these problems, but it introduces others. Parents may not remember exactly when their child achieved certain milestones of development. They may be so concerned about worrisome behaviors that they forget the milestones the child does meet. Parents may also be so distressed about the child's odd behaviors that they have trouble thinking and talking about them. Most assessment teams use both methods to overcome these pitfalls. They observe the child's behavior and they ask parents about current behavior and developmental history. Although it may seem redundant, this combination of methods helps ensure getting the most valid picture of the child.

Until the last decade or two, the only way to diagnose autism was for a clinician, usually a medical doctor or a psychologist, to see the child and talk with the parents, engaging the child in some informal interaction and informally interviewing the parents. These clinicians used their experience to judge whether the information gathered in these informal sessions justified a diagnosis of autism, comparing their observations and interview outcomes with diagnostic criteria in the most current diagnostic manual. Several standard instruments have been developed since the early 2000s, however, to accomplish behavior observation and parent report. These instruments have been refined by testing their effectiveness in trials involving large numbers of children and comparing the instruments' findings with the judgments of experienced professionals. These standardized protocols allow a wider range of professionals to contribute to diagnostic decisions and make research on these conditions more valid because children are identified the same way, regardless of where they live or how experienced the testing clinician may be.

Standardized Assessment

The Autism Diagnostic Observation Schedule (ADOS; Lord et al., 2012) is perhaps the most widely used direct observation method. This is not a test, but a protocol for observation that engages the child in a series of activities, such as playing with balls, bubbles, and shape sorters. Minor frustrations, called *presses,* however, are introduced in the course of this play. For example, the examiner occasionally covers up the holes in the shape sorter or removes the bubble blower when the child is engaged with it. These presses are inserted in order to elicit social interactions, which may be difficult for the child with ASD to muster. The ADOS has several modules for children at different developmental levels, as indexed by how much speech they produce. The Toddler Module is designed to be used with children from 12 to 30 months with little use of words. Module 1 is aimed at children with some words but few phrases in their speech. Children who use some phrases but do not consistently use full sentences are administered Module 2. Module 3 is for children who are verbally fluent, whereas Module 4 is used with adolescents and adults who are verbally fluent. Each module takes about an hour to administer and contains several sets of activities that include play or construction, interaction with books and stories, imitation or use of gestures, as well as activities suited to the developmental level of the module's target audience. The Toddler Module includes pretending to bathe an infant, Modules 1 and 2 include enacting a birthday party, and Modules 3 and 4 include having conversations about friendship and loneliness. Children are given points during the ADOS for showing behaviors characteristic of ASD so that the more atypical behaviors a child shows, the more points the child earns. Cut-off scores are established for each module that indicate when the child meets criteria for ASD. A lot of research has gone into developing the ADOS and shows that it is quite accurate, relative to experienced clinical judgment, in recognizing autism in children at a range of developmental levels. The ADOS has an accompanying parent report form, the Autism Diagnostic Interview–Revised (ADI-R; Rutter, LeConteur, & Lord, 2003). It's quite lengthy and detailed, taking about 2 hours to administer. It may be used in conjunction with the ADOS observation to make or validate a diagnostic decision.

There are a few other behavior observation protocols for young children that are aimed at identifying ASD—the Autism Observation Scale for Infants (AOSI; Bryson, Zwaigenbaum, McDermott, Rombough, & Brian, 2008) and the Early Social Communication Scales (Mundy et al., 2003). Some insurance companies, birth-to-3 agencies, or school-based programs may have regulations or guidelines about what diagnostic procedure has to be used in order for a child to qualify for services or reimbursement. Although the *DSM-5* (American Psychiatric Association, 2013) criteria are generally used by medical professionals to make diagnoses, schools and birth-to-3 agencies may have somewhat different criteria. The bottom line is that a formal diagnosis must be made by a medical professional, psychologist, or educational team in order to receive services for ASD. Although use of a formal protocol for the diagnosis is not always required, and medical professionals are likely to directly apply the criteria in Box 1.1 to their observations without using any specified protocol for observation, most educational teams will employ some kind of standard method, such as the ADOS (Lord et al., 2012) or AOSI. If your child is involved in a research study, then the ADOS and ADI-R (Rutter et al., 2003) are likely to be used to qualify your child for participation.

WHAT'S THE DIFFERENCE BETWEEN SCREENING AND DIAGNOSIS?

If you or your doctor suspects ASD, then there is usually a step to be taken before requesting a full-blown evaluation. This step is called *screening*. Screening is a brief assessment aimed at finding children who show some red flags for developmental difficulty and may be in need of a more comprehensive assessment to determine whether they have a developmental disorder and the type of disorder. There are two kinds of screening. Universal or population-based screening provides a brief assessment to everyone in a population. For example, many school systems hold kindergarten screenings before children enter school to identify if any of the 5-year-olds show signs of developmental delay. If so, these children will be referred for more in-depth assessment by the special education team. Pediatricians are encouraged by their professional organization to do universal screening for ASD at all 18- or 24-month well-baby checkups, but this recommendation, unfortunately, is not always followed.

The second kind of screening occurs when there is a suspicion that a particular child may be experiencing a developmental problem. Even if your child's pediatrician does not do universal screening for ASD, he or she may be able to provide screening in the office if there are concerns about the child's development or if you request it. If the screen is positive, then a referral for a complete evaluation can be made to a birth-to-3 agency. Table 1.1 lists some of the instruments commonly used as screeners for ASD. It's important to remember, though, that these screening instruments are not sufficient in themselves to make a diagnosis of ASD. Identification by way of a screening interview or questionnaire should always be followed by a more in-depth diagnostic assessment that examines a child's cognitive, social, motor, and communication skills and includes an observation of behavior.

What Happens at a Diagnostic Assessment?

If your child is younger than 3 years old, then chances are that a diagnostic assessment will take place in your home. One or several people may come to do testing, interviews, and observation, and they will usually bring materials with them, like those the team brought to Mariana's home. You may be asked to bring your child to a testing center at a school or other community facility, however, if your child is older than 3 years old. Wherever the assessment takes place, there are a few things you will want to keep in mind.

- Any young child can look worse one day than another. If your child isn't able to show the examiners everything he or she is able to do, then remember that you can fill in the gaps during your interviews with the assessors. Evaluators know parents are the best reporters on their child's behavior and will take seriously any information you add to what they are able to observe themselves.

- The assessment is likely to last longer than your child is at his or her best. The evaluators generally have a good deal of experience working with young

Table 1.1.   Screening instruments for autism in young children

Screener	Age range
Brief Infant-Toddler Social and Emotional Assessment (BITSEA) (Briggs-Gowan & Carter, 2006)	12–35 months
Childhood Autism Rating Scale (CARS) (Schopler, Reichler, & Renner, 1988)	2 years +
Early Screening of Autistic Traits (ESAT) (Dietz, Swinkel, van Daalen, van Engeland, & Buitelaar, 2006)	13–23 months
First Year Inventory (Resnick, Baranek, Reavis, Watson, & Crais, 2007)	12 months
Gilliam Autism Rating Scales (Gilliam, 2006)	3–22 months
Infant-Toddler Checklist (Wetherby & Prizant, 2003)	9–24 months
Modified Checklist for Autism in Toddlers (M-CHAT) (Robins & Dumont-Mathieu, 2006)	16–45 months
Pervasive Developmental Disorders Screening Test–II (Siegel, 2004)	12–48 months
Screening Tool for Autism in Two-Year-Olds (STAT) (Stone, Conrood, Turner, & Pozdol, 2004)	14–36 months
Social Communication Questionnaire (SCQ) (Rutter, Bailey, & Lord, 2003)	4 years +

children and they know that children get tired. If your child seems to do better in some parts of the assessment than others, then be sure to tell the examiners if something looks to you like atypical behavior for him or her. Don't worry if your child tends to wind down toward the end of a long evaluation. Examiners usually understand that this is expected and interpret their observations accordingly.

- The evaluators are trying to get a snapshot of what your child is like today. They aren't projecting today's behavior into the future. In fact, many of the assessments used with young children are known to be unreliable for predicting later performance, and the scores your child gets now don't necessarily foretell how well he or she will do at school age. What the evaluators need to find out is what developmentally appropriate skills the child has trouble with now so those skills can be supported through instruction and guided practice in an intervention program over the next few months and years. The aim of all early intervention is not to permanently identify children as having ASD or any other disability but to provide supports that maximize children's ability to acquire age-appropriate skills in the early years when children are most malleable to see how far they can go.

- Although it is hard to watch your child struggle with tasks, it is really to everyone's advantage that the evaluation shows both what he or she can and cannot do. Educators can't help your child unless they understand all strengths and weaknesses. If they only see the strengths, then they may miss important areas that need instruction or support. Although you want your child's strengths to be visible, and you can certainly tell the evaluator if you see your child behaving in a way that is not typical of him or her, the evaluators need to get a glimpse of what is really hard or uninteresting to your child so they can plan the most appropriate program. Although all parents have a natural impulse to want to show children at their best, seeing both the highs and the lows in this situation is what will help your child the most.

How Will My Child Be Assessed? The content of the diagnostic assessment will vary from agency to agency, but, in general, the following areas will be addressed.

Behaviors Symptomatic of ASD Usually a combination of direct observation, parent report, and structured instruments, such as the ADOS (Lord et al., 2012) and ADI-R (Rutter et al., 2003), will be used to look for the presence of symptoms of ASD.

Cognition The assessment usually will include a measure of cognitive development, or thinking/problem-solving skills. Tests for young children involve doing puzzles, imitating designs with blocks, simple drawing, stacking blocks or rings, finding toys hidden under things, matching objects or pictures, and so forth. Again, you may see your child being asked to do things that are challenging or just beyond current abilities. Remember that the examiners need to keep asking your child to do harder items until he or she reaches the point where several items in a row are failed. It's very common for children to be able to do some harder items and not others, and the examiner needs to continue presenting tasks until the child can't do any of them. Although it may be hard to see your child fail, try to remember that the examiners want to see how far he or she can go and don't want to stop providing an opportunity to show what he or she can do until they are sure the highest level has been reached. The only way to get there is to keep going until he or she fails consistently. Although it may be painful to watch the child being asked to do things he or she can't do, you will want your child to get credit for going as far as possible on the test.

Verbal Skills Many tests of cognition have one scale for nonverbal skills, such as those we just described, and another for verbal skills, such as recognizing words, naming objects, and following simple directions. That's because some children (and many with ASD) can be quite good at one of these kinds of skills but not good at the other. For example, it's quite common to see young children with age-appropriate skills in nonverbal puzzles and tasks but delays in talking and understanding language. Evaluators will want to know whether your child functions at age level in both kinds of tasks and, if not, whether one is a relative strength. They may use a test with both verbal and nonverbal scales, or they may use a separate test that was specially designed to focus on speech-language and communication skills. Some of the tests commonly used to assess speech-language and communication in young children are listed in Table 1.2.

Motor Skills Much of early child development involves learning to accomplish large motor activities, such as sitting up, crawling, walking, jumping, hopping, and climbing stairs, as well as small motor skills, such as grasping, picking things up, passing things from hand to hand, holding and using crayons and pencils, and stringing beads. These motor skills enable more cognitive achievements by allowing the child to get to objects to explore them, to manipulate objects in a wide range of ways, and to see how objects fit and work together. Many children with ASD show relative strengths in motor skills, so this may be a way for evaluators to observe some of the child's higher levels of function. They will probably ask your child to jump, hop, climb stairs, draw a line, string a bead, and so forth in order to assess this area. If your child does not demonstrate skills you've seen in other situations, then the examiners can take your report into account.

Self-Help and Adaptive Skills It's one thing to develop motor and verbal skills, but another to use them to accomplish day-to-day activities. Children with ID sometimes show relative strengths in their ability to accomplish daily living tasks, such as dressing, bathing, feeding themselves, getting around the community, and doing chores. Self-care skills are often less developed than other

Table 1.2. Specialized tests commonly used to assess speech-language and communication in young children

Test	Description
Communication and Symbolic Behavior Scales Developmental Profile (CSBS DP™) (Wetherby & Prizant, 2002)	Includes assessment of symbolic play, nonverbal communication, and expressive and receptive language; requires videotaped observation; accompanied by parent report form
Language Development Survey (LDS) (Rescorla, 1989)	Parent report of expressive vocabulary size; good validity on identifying language delay in toddlers
The MacArthur-Bates Communicative Development Inventories User's Guide and Technical Manual, Second Edition (CDI) (Fenson et al., 2006)	Parent report instrument with scales for assessing expressive and receptive vocabulary sizes and early grammatical production; often used in research studies
Preschool Language Scale—Fifth Edition (PLS-5) (Zimmerman, Steiner, & Pond, 2011)	Measures receptive and expressive language skills; provides standard scores and percentile ranks in addition to age equivalents
Receptive-Expressive Emergent Language Scale—Third Edition (REEL-3) (Bzoch, League, & Brown, 2003)	Administered through a combination of structured interview and direct observation; tends to overestimate comprehension
Rossetti Infant and Toddler Language Scale (Rossetti, 1990)	Used to assess preverbal and verbal communication skills and interaction; looks at language comprehension, language expression, interaction, attachment, gestures, pragmatics, and play
Reynell Developmental Language Scales III (Edwards et al., 1999)	Verbal comprehension scale measures receptive language skills (both verbal and nonverbal); the expressive language scale assesses expressive language skills using items that test sentence structure, vocabulary, and sentence meaning
Sequenced Inventory of Communication Development—Revised (SICD-R) (Hedrick, Prather, & Tobin, 1995)	Measures preverbal and verbal skills in expressive and receptive modalities
Test of Early Language Development—Third Edition (TELD-3) (Hresko, Reid, & Hamill, 1999)	Includes scores for subtests of receptive and expressive language; shows reliability, validity, and limited bias

areas in many children with ASD, however, even in those with strong cognitive and verbal skills. Adaptive skills are crucial to the ability to attain some level of self-sufficiency, so it is important that they be part of an intervention program. Learning age-appropriate self-help skills sets a child on a path toward independence, and it's never too early to start, especially because children with ASD may take longer to learn these skills than their peers. Self-help generally is assessed through parent interviews or questionnaires because the child cannot be expected to exhibit skills such as dressing and bathing during an assessment. There are several standardized interviews and questionnaires designed to evaluate development in the self-help area.

Table 1.3 lists some of the most commonly used general assessment instruments for young children and identifies which aspects of behavior they are designed to evaluate so you can be familiar with the tools used in your child's assessment.

WHAT'S THE DIFFERENCE BETWEEN A MEDICAL AND AN EDUCATIONAL DIAGNOSIS?

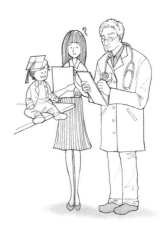

A medical diagnosis can only be made by a medical professional. In states that mandate insurance coverage for services for children with ASD, you may be required to obtain a medical diagnosis in order to obtain insurance coverage. Medical diagnosis entails an evaluation by a physician, usually a pediatrician, child neurologist, or child psychiatrist (some states include psychologists in this category), who will usually observe your child and interview parents in order to compare the findings to the *DSM*-5 (American Psychiatric Association, 2013) criteria. A medical diagnosis may not be necessary, however, to obtain services that are provided by a birth-to-3 agency or preschool or school program. If your birth-to-3 or school team evaluates your child, then they may confer an educational diagnosis, meaning that the child meets the local agency's criteria as assessed by trained educational professionals and can be provided with services under this educational assessment. The

Table 1.3. Commonly used assessment instruments for young children

Measure	Area assessed	For more information
Assessment, Evaluation, and Programming System for Infants and Children (AEPS®), Second Edition, Volumes 1–4 (Bricker et al., 2002)	Fine motor, gross motor, cognitive, adaptive, social-communication, social	http://www.aepsinteractive.com
Bayley Scales of Infant and Toddler Development, Third Edition (BSID-III) (Bayley, 2005)	Cognitive, motor, language, social-emotional, adaptive	http://www.psychometrics.cam.ac.uk/services/psychometric-tests/bayley-scales
Battelle Developmental Inventory, Second Edition (BDI–2) (Newborg, Stock, Wnek, Guidubaldi, & Svinicki, 2002)	Adaptive, language, motor, cognitive	http://learningdisabilities.about.com/od/intelligencetests/p/battelledevelop.htm
Brigance Inventory of Early Development (IED III), Early Childhood Edition (Brigance, Bellerica, MA: Curriculum Associates, 2013)	Motor, self-help, language, social-emotional development	http://www.curriculumassociates.com/products/detail.aspx?title=BrigEC-IED3-sum
Early Learning Accomplishment Profile (Early-LAP/ELAP) (Glover, Preminger, & Sanford, 2002)	Motor, cognitive, language, self-help, social-emotional	http://ectacenter.org/~pdfs/eco/LAP_crosswalk_10-3-06.pdf
Mullen Scales of Early Learning (MSEL) (Mullen, 1995)	Cognitive, language, motor	http://www.ecasd.k12.wi.us/student_services/assessments/MSEL-AGS.pdf
Transdisciplinary Play-Based Assessment, Second Edition (TPBA2) (Linder, 2008)	Cognitive, social-emotional, communication and language, sensorimotor	http://brookespublishing.com/tpba2

criteria for medical and educational diagnoses are usually pretty similar. The main difference is who does the evaluation; a medical professional is required for the medical diagnosis, whereas educators working as a team who are trained to assess ASD can provide an educational diagnosis. If insurance coverage is not an issue, then you may not need a medical diagnosis and your educational team's assessment may be adequate to make your child eligible for publicly-funded services. It's important to understand that the medical diagnosis is no more valid than the educational one in most cases, and if you are satisfied with the assessment and treatment plan provided by your local birth-to-3 agency or school, then it is not absolutely necessary to seek diagnosis from a medical expert. You would need to obtain a medical opinion only if you have concerns about the results of your child's assessment or if insurance coverage is an issue.

WHAT DOES THIS DIAGNOSIS MEAN FOR OUR CHILD AND FAMILY OVER THE NEXT FEW YEARS?

If your child has recently been diagnosed with ASD, then you are probably going through a difficult time in your life. You are facing many decisions about how to handle the situation right now and many worries about what it means for the future. If you have other children, then you are probably concerned about what it will mean for them. If you don't have other children, then you may be wondering whether to have more children. All these worries place extra pressure on parents at a time when they are feeling the need to learn a huge amount about ASD, how to treat it, and about their local service system, as well as a need to explain the situation to friends and family. Parents may also feel the pressure to immediately find the most effective, comprehensive services for their child, to cover the costs of assessments and treatments, and to adjust to this new, frightening reality in their lives. Nothing we can say can change any of these feelings. What we will try to do is to share our combined 50 years of experience in working with children with ASD and their families to help you navigate this challenging time.

One of the hardest things about learning that you have a child with a disability is that there is no well-trodden path for you to follow. For every other important life event—birth, marriage, and even death—there are customs and rituals dictated by culture to provide guidance about how to feel and behave. Brides are "blushing"; babies are "bundles of joy"; death is seen differently across cultures, but all provide some form of understanding and some set of ritual activities to help people through times of loss. Communities have rites that provide support and validation for other life events, such as weddings, graduations, and funerals. There are no culturally established ways to deal with learning that you have a child with a disability. There is no common language, no prescribed activities or gatherings, and no customary way for friends and family to help. This lack of communally sanctioned reactions leaves everyone—not just you but your family, friends, and neighbors—feeling adrift, and you may feel alone because others often do not know how to be helpful and supportive.

There is no easy solution to this problem, but reaching out to families in the same situation is one strategy. Besides providing emotional support, they may already have learned a lot of what you feel you need to know and can help you identify local resources, educational services, experienced medical providers, places you can comfortably take your child with ASD, and baby sitters who can handle children with disabilities, as well as tricks they've learned to help manage difficult situations. Because there is no ready-made community for families of children with disabilities, it's important for your family's overall well-being to begin to form one for yourselves. Web-based resources for finding other families of children with ASD are provided in the Suggested Resources appendix, but you will also want to discover local sources of support.

It is important to remember that there is no right way to respond. Some parents will feel relieved to have a name for a problem that seemed mysterious, whereas others will be angry. Some may feel a new sense of energy and purpose in finding the best solutions for their child's problem, whereas others will feel immobilized and in shock. However you feel is exactly the way you should feel. What can be hard is that sometimes two parents will have different responses to the news about the child they share. One may feel suspicious that the diagnosis is incorrect and want more opinions and assessments, whereas the other may feel the diagnosis confirms lingering fears and wants to move forward to get a program started. Negotiating this as a couple can have its own challenges. It sometimes helps to remember that we are each entitled to our individual reactions and those reactions are going to vary from person to person. Each of us has to work our way through our instinctive reactions to find ways to cope; the soundest strategy is to help each other find a way forward that works for everyone involved. It helps to remember that initial responses don't last forever. Feelings will change as more knowledge and social support is developed and as the child begins making progress.

What can your family expect over the next years as you face the future with your child with ASD? The first thing to expect is that things will change. Your child will grow and learn as every child does, perhaps not at the same pace, but you will see progress. It is reasonable to be optimistic about the potential for improvement, especially in the years before your child turns 6 or 7 years old. For example, research shows that the majority of children with ASD who aren't talking at age 2 or 3 do begin using speech by school age. Their speech may not be perfect, but 80% of children with ASD will develop speech skills that are adequate to communicate basic wants and needs. There is reason to be hopeful, especially with early intervention in place.

Other symptoms will change over time, too. Some children who are very withdrawn during the preschool years become more open to social overtures. Some who are very active as preschoolers grow calmer and mellower with time. It is hard to predict the degree and direction of change, but you can be virtually certain that change will happen. If there are symptoms that are especially distressing to you and your family, it is important to talk with your educational team about focusing on them and making sure that they change as rapidly as possible, even if it means making other important skills a lower priority. If you only have so many hours of applied behavior analysis (ABA) allotted to your child's program, and you are very concerned about toilet training, then it makes sense to ask your ABA providers to organize their hours so that toilet training can get the maximal amount of programming. Once it is achieved, hours can always be allocated in a different way. If your child is not communicating and is using other, maladaptive behaviors such as head-banging to express frustration or other needs, then you may want to increase time spent on communication skills and decrease some other services until more adaptive ways to get ideas across are learned. Things will certainly change, and one of your goals during the early years is to try to channel that change in a direction that makes your child function as well as possible within your family.

If your child is receiving birth-to-3 services, then you can expect those services to continue until the third birthday, but there will be a transition to a school-based program at that time. Rather than taking place in your home or child care center, the school program will be housed in a facility managed by the local education agency (LEA) and will include other children with and without disabilities. It will probably be held 4–5 days per week from 2.5 to 6 hours per day, just like a regular school program. The school will usually provide transportation as well as programming, so your child may be out of the home for a majority of the day and may be quite tired when he or she returns home. Some children may nap, but others may be irritable and agitated when tired, so it is a good idea to plan a snack and some relaxing, enjoyable activities (e.g., watching their favorite shows, playing computer games) for at least a short time after school or preschool. Many families benefit from hiring a family helper, such as a teenage neighbor who comes to the home after school to play with and oversee the child with ASD and provides the child with a safe time to relax after the school day. This can allow parents some quiet time to prepare dinner or help other children with homework without having to supervise or entertain the child with ASD.

There will be difficult times, when you feel overwhelmed by your child's needs and by efforts to balance them with the needs of others in the family. But you will find moments of joy with your child with ASD, just as you would with any child. You will feel proud when he or she says a first word, completes a first puzzle, or gets through a whole therapy session without a tantrum. Although children with ASD don't always demonstrate affection the way other children do, you will learn to recognize the unique ways in which your child shows how important you are to him or her and will find deep satisfaction in discovering them.

Being the parent of a child with ASD is not a job anyone volunteers for, but becoming a parent never comes with any guarantees. Parents of typically developing children can suffer heartache over bad choices their children make, diseases they succumb to, or opportunities of which they fail to take advantage. The most important consideration for parents of a child with ASD is to find a way to accept who the child is and find ways to treasure what is exceptional about your child. Although, you will want the most comprehensive, effective educational program possible for your child, it is important to remember, that no educational program is going to turn a child into someone he or she is not or change a child's fundamental nature.

Children with ASD have personalities, just like other children, and those personalities are an aspect of who they are, independent of their disabilities. Some are curious; some are sensitive; some are enthusiastic; some are highly active; some quiet. You wouldn't want to change those temperamental characteristics of a typical child (and you probably couldn't, even if you tried), and you won't change them fundamentally in your child with ASD either. A good program can reduce maladaptive behaviors, increase positive ones, and teach important new skills. But it can't make a child with ASD into a different person. Even the 10% or so of children who showed symptoms of ASD as youngsters but had optimum outcomes that place them outside the autism spectrum by school age tended to retain problems with using language in social contexts (Fein et al., 2013; Kelley, Paul, Fein, & Naigles, 2006) that colored their personal interaction style. These "optimal outcomes" will not be available to every child, no matter how hard you work to provide the best program possible. The great majority of young children with ASD will grow to be older children and adults with ASD. The best things we can do for them are to provide the highest level of educational and behavior support we can, and to appreciate their individuality, because children with ASD are as distinct and unique as every other human being.

The challenges and sorrows that come with having a child with ASD cannot be sugarcoated. We would be lying if we said you will never have hard times. With the help of others, though, you can find a way to create the educational opportunities your child needs and still experience the joys of being a family when you are armed with knowledge of your child's condition, empathy for the child as well as for the other members of your family who share your struggles, and an appreciation of the unique viewpoint from which your child sees the world.

The opportunities for people with ASD are more varied and open today than they were in the mid-2000s. Growing public interest in and awareness of the syndrome means almost everyone knows about ASD. That means you don't have to feel embarrassed if your child has a tantrum in the supermarket—you can just explain to the other shoppers, "My child has autism," knowing that most people will understand. It also means there are many changes taking place in society for all people with disabilities, but perhaps most intensely for people with ASD, to accommodate and include people with all kinds of challenges in our communities. For example, there are efforts to devise programs to aid the transition from school to work for young adults with ASD and provide vocational training and opportunities in mainstream employment. In addition, there are specialized independent living programs, college programs, and recreational programs for people with ASD. Governmental agencies are awakening (with a lot of push from families) to their responsibilities to provide funding for programs that make mainstream participation possible. By the time your child is ready to take part in these programs, there is good reason to be optimistic that there will be a broader menu of services and supports for your family to consider than there are today.

What Are the Characteristics of Young Children with Autism Spectrum Disorder?

Chapter 1 reviewed some of the assessment procedures used to identify young children with ASD as well as some of the characteristic behaviors that evaluators are looking for to make a diagnosis. Yet that is a somewhat different question from asking

- What are young children with ASD like?

- How do they behave?

- What do they like and not like to do?

- What do they need from their families?

- What are they like as teenagers?

- What will they do when they grow up?

Truthfully, you don't know the answers to these questions when you bring a newborn home from the hospital, so you won't know them for your child with ASD either, before or after he or she receives a diagnosis. Every child with ASD is unique, just like every child in the world. This is true for children who have all kinds of disabilities as well as children who develop typically. It is even more true in the case of ASD, though, because it is a spectrum disorder with a wide range of expression. ASD can appear as an extremely mild impairment that may seem like a quirk rather than a disability or as a very severe impairment that limits all aspects of cognitive, social, and language development. So it isn't really possible to describe what a typical child with ASD will be like. Although there are a range of general profiles seen in children with ASD, no child is going to conform exactly to any of these patterns.

> *Just remember, no child is going to conform exactly to any of these patterns.*

LOW- VERSUS HIGH-FUNCTIONING ASD

Connor and Ben have just started kindergarten in an inclusive public school. Both boys have been diagnosed with ASD, but they are very different. Connor is described as having high-functioning ASD (HFA) and Ben as having low-functioning ASD (LFA). Connor is highly verbal, loves asking adults questions, and loves to read. He reads at a second-grade level but doesn't always understand what he reads. During circle time he will read what's on the walls, including safety and fire notices. He also reads his parents' letters and bills when they are left out, and he will read notices on trucks when he is in the car. He sometimes uses this as an avoidance technique when asked to do something he doesn't want to do. Connor also has difficulty adjusting to changes in routine and being flexible. He tends to be quite rigid. When students in Connor's class were asked to copy a picture of a face, Connor's teacher complimented him on his drawing and said, "Connor, this is great! It looks just the same as mine; it's a match!" Connor became very upset and started to cry, "It's not the same! It's not great! It's not a match!" He took his picture and tore it up. He recognized that the pictures were not identical and this upset him.

Ben, who had also completed the picture, responded quite differently. When his teacher complimented him and said, "Great picture, Ben!" he smiled without looking at the teacher, twirled his fingers with excitement, and said, "Great picture, Ben!" Although Ben is described as having LFA because he has limited speech and is not as as academically successful as Connor, he is able to adjust more easily to changes in the school routine and is more easily able to cope with various events and interactions throughout the school day. Here is another example of how the two boys are different.

Changes in the schedule are quite typical in a kindergarten classroom—a teacher may be absent or the daily routine may need to be changed. Ben adjusts well when he is shown the change on his individual visual schedule. If it is raining, Ben doesn't mind if recess is indoors instead of on the playground. Connor, though, gets very upset when his teacher is absent and will repeatedly ask about her whereabouts. He worries that something serious may be wrong. He also does not easily adjust to missed playground time and will stand by the classroom daily schedule and repeat, "11:10. Go outside to the playground." He is also known to act out when these changes in his routine happen, and it can take the entire school day for him to settle down. Although Connor is highly verbal, he is unable to express these frustrations in words. His rigidity and difficulty thinking flexibly make it hard for him to adjust to changes in his routine. Connor is doing well academically, but his social challenges and difficulty being flexible make it really hard for him at times and affect how he functions in the classroom. Ben does not use as much language and has fewer academic skills, but he responds to changes in the classroom by using his personal visual schedule and is able to tolerate these changes. The teacher has to differentiate her instruction for Ben and Connor. Although both boys have ASD, they need varying degrees of support.

As we said, professionals working with children with ASD generally divide the population into two categories—low and high functioning. A lot of parents don't like this designation because it seems to imply something uncomplimentary about the low-functioning group, but the designation is meant to describe the degree to which the child is likely to require supports and services in a school setting and is not meant to stigmatize children who function at a lower level.

In many disorders, this kind of categorization is done with terms that describe the severity of the disorder (e.g., mild, moderate, profound), but this system doesn't work well for people with ASD because a person could have a very severe form of autism that would profoundly affect the ability to get along in the world in the presence of very high intelligence and certain kinds of academic achievement. The low- and high-functioning distinction is likely to continue to be used until there's a better way to describe the level of need a person with ASD has for supportive services.

The difference between LFA and HFA is generally seen in the level of cognitive and language function an individual shows. People who score below the cutoff for intellectual disability (ID) on an IQ test (around 70–75) are usually considered to have an ID. This used to be called *mental retardation,* a term now considered outdated. People with ASD may have ID that co-occurs with their autism. This means they score below 70 on an IQ test and have symptoms of ASD, including impairments in social interaction and communication as well

> The designation is meant to describe the degree to which the child is likely to require supports and services in a school setting and is not meant to stigmatize children who function at a lower level.

as restricted and repetitive behaviors. Individuals who show this profile of low IQ scores combined with symptoms of autism tend to be labeled as low-functioning autism (LFA), especially if they show limited speech. Those who score above 70 on an IQ test and have at least some use of speech, even if it is delayed for their age, are typically considered to have high-functioning autism (HFA). Of course, there will be some individuals who fall in a gray area, with IQs below 70 but useable speech or higher nonverbal IQs but extremely limited speech. There is tremendous variability in the severity of social-communication impairment and repetitive behavior in both the LFA and HFA groups. Children generally are not designated as LFA or HFA until they reach school age because there can be significant growth in cognitive and language skills during the preschool years, and many children with ASD do not acquire functional speech until the end of the preschool or beginning of the school-age period. Discussion regarding the LFA and HFA distinction needs to wait until autism in the school years is described. For now, let's start from the beginning.

WHAT ARE CHILDREN WITH ASD LIKE?

In this section, we will describe how ASD can appear at various stages in development from infancy through adolescence. Although, again, each child will develop in a unique way, there are general trends that are often seen as children with ASD grow.

Infants with ASD

In the last decade there has been a great deal of interest in what ASD looks like in the first year of life, primarily because it is hoped that if the syndrome can be identified earlier, then some of its consequences may be averted. Despite the fact that ASD has been recognized since the mid-1940s, little is known about how it emerges in the first year or so of life because almost no children are identified as having it at these early ages. Children with ASD often look very typical during their first year. They don't have any physical differences that allow the syndrome to be recognized. The behavior of most children who end up with the diagnosis doesn't seem unusual in the first months of life. Unlike children with ID, those with ASD often achieve motor milestones, such as rolling over, sitting up, and crawling, more or less at the expected time.

Sally Ozonoff and her colleagues (2010) reported that behavioral signs of autism are not usually evident at birth or in the first 6 months of life. Instead, these researchers observed a pattern of development in which key social-communication behaviors that ordinarily emerge toward the end of the first year of life, such as looking at what others look at or point to and coordinating smiling and looking with babbling, were diminished relative to typical peers in children who went on to be diagnosed with ASD, and these behaviors became more atypical as the children moved through the second year of life. Again, not every child with ASD shows this pattern; some parents of children with ASD recall that their infants were unusually quiet, or inconsolable, or didn't like to be cuddled, but it is true that children with ASD can look perfectly average during much of the first year and then seem to become stalled in development or even regress during their second year. This is likely because the hallmarks of ASD, the social-communication behaviors that allow infants to begin initiating communication and maintaining others' attention, begin to unfold between 6 and 12 months and are critical milestones of development during the second year. There may be subtle differences in the first months of life that adults just don't notice.

Hallmarks of ASD, the social-communication behaviors that allow infants to begin initiating communication and maintaining others' attention, begin to unfold between 6 and 12 months and are critical milestones of development during the second year.

Or, social-communication demands just don't stress the system very much in the first months because adults do almost all the work in starting interactions and keeping them going with infants under 6 months of age. If only these systems are impaired, as is true for some but not all children with ASD, then there may be very little in the way of red flags during the first months of life.

Toddlers with ASD

Leo is 18 months old and has an older brother diagnosed with ASD. His parents had been keeping a close eye on him and hadn't really noticed anything to be concerned about until just after Leo's first birthday. He seemed to be following the typical pattern of development and was using a few words to ask for items he wanted, such as juice or chips, by his first birthday. Unlike his brother with ASD, he was not a fussy eater and he did not have difficulty making the transition from one place to another.

But his parents noticed some changes in Leo's behavior after his first birthday. Leo would take his brother's plastic elephants and line them up in the hallway, in his bedroom, and in the car. He liked being cuddled, which they initially thought was a good sign, but they noticed that Leo would go up to people he didn't know very well, sit on their lap, and stroke the skin of their necks. They also noticed that Leo would sing most of the day rather than using his words to talk. When he would see his mother when she came back from work he would greet her by singing, "No more monkeys jumping on the bed" as this is what they sang at night. Leo's parents knew that these changes were possible red flags and they spoke to his brother's SLP, who suggested Leo have an assessment.

The signs of ASD become noticeable in many children around their first birthday. Geraldine Dawson and her colleagues (2010) looked at videotapes of first birthday parties of children who were later diagnosed with ASD. They found that by 12 months of age, these infants showed less ability to share attention to objects with others (by looking at what others looked at or pointed to), were less likely to look at others' faces, showed less smiling and pointing, and were less likely to respond to their names. They found that professionals could often identify which 12-month-olds would be diagnosed with ASD in the future. Videotapes of younger infants (8–10 months of age) showed similar trends, but professionals were less able to identify affected children at these earlier ages.

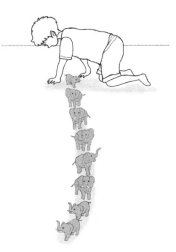

Although ASD is sometimes not diagnosed until age 3 or 4, parents often become concerned during a child's second year as he or she begins to look different from other toddlers. One difference parents notice is that children with ASD often are much slower to acquire speech. First words are very often delayed; when they emerge, new words are learned slowly and word combinations take a long time to appear. Some children may start to say a few words, then become stuck and don't progress in their language development. Others may stop using words they previously used and go back to being nonverbal. Parents often worry about this kind of regression in toddlers, but studies looking at toddlers who showed regression found that their outcomes were not very different from toddlers with ASD who did not show regression (Shumway et al., 2011).

Children with ASD often are much slower to acquire speech.

In addition to not talking, parents of toddlers diagnosed with ASD also notice that their children don't listen. Whereas typically developing children begin responding to their name as early as 6 months of age, children with ASD often do not answer to their names until the toddler and preschool years. These children also tend to respond less reliably to talk of any kind. Sometimes their parents suspect they are deaf. When hearing testing shows no loss of sensitivity to sound, these children are often referred for the developmental evaluation that identifies ASD.

Parents of toddlers diagnosed with ASD also notice that their children don't listen. These children also tend to respond less reliably to talk of any kind.

Apart from a slow or interrupted course of language learning, toddlers with ASD also don't use the other means of communication that typically developing children use. They don't point to things they want others to look at, show things they like to others, look at things and then at people to get people to see what they see, or try to get others' attention with babbling.

That's not to say that toddlers with ASD don't communicate at all. They can be quite insistent in trying to get others to do or get things for them, but they tend not to use usual gestures such as pointing, sounds such as babbling, or gaze. Instead, they may make unusual sounds, such as squeals or grunts, or grab an adult's hand without looking at his or her face to get help.

That's not to say that toddlers with ASD don't communicate at all. They may make unusual sounds, such as squeals or grunts, or grab an adult's hand without looking at his or her face to get help.

Toddlers with ASD will sometimes begin to show other unusual behaviors such as unusual postures of their arms or hands, holding objects at odd angles and peering at them, or taking an intense interest in parts of objects, such as wheels, rather than the whole object. They may also find enjoyment in repetitive activities, such as repeatedly making toys in a "Poppin' Pals" pop up. Sometimes the repetitive activities they like will involve unusual objects that wouldn't normally be thought of as toys, such as rubber bands they like to twang repeatedly. Or they may enjoy repetitive bodily motions, such as spinning.

Some toddlers with ASD begin to show unusual sensitivities, such as exaggerated responses to certain noises, lights, foods, or textures. Other children may be insensitive to things that would bother most other people. The source of these sensory differences is still a mystery, and not all children with ASD have them. Typically developing toddlers, too, sometimes show the same kinds of sensitivities, at least for a time. What to do about these sensitivities is also a matter of debate. It's tempting to try to protect the child with increased sensitivity from the problem stimulation (e.g., running the vacuum cleaner only when the child is out of the house). Sensory integration and other sensory-oriented therapies have been proposed, but there isn't a lot of evidence that they actually improve children's ability to process sensory stimuli. Lucker (2013) argued that systematic desensitization is the best approach to reduce these issues. Families can start by providing a version of the stimulus the child can tolerate (such as recording the vacuum cleaner sound and playing it back at a volume turned down low while pretending to run the vacuum cleaner with the power off) and gradually increasing the intensity of the stimulus a little bit at a time.

Several resources are available for learning about what autism looks like in the toddler years for families who are beginning to have concerns about their children. Autism Speaks, a nonprofit organization, provides a video glossary of early symptoms:

http://www.autismspeaks.org/what-autism/video-glossary

The Kennedy Krieger Institute also provides tutorial videos on early signs of ASD:

http://www.kennedykrieger.org/patient-care/patient-care-centers/center-autism
    -and-related-disorders/outreach-training/early-signs-of-autism-video
    -tutorial

The First Signs website provides additional information.

http://www.firstsigns.org/concerns/flags.htm

http://www.firstsigns.org/asd_video_glossary/asdvg_about.htm

Preschoolers with ASD

Typically developing preschoolers acquire their language, communication, and play skills in a relatively standard sequence. Although children with ASD usually acquire skills such as sitting, walking, and crawling in the typical order, their language, social-communication, and play skills will unfold in a more unusual way. The differences seen in toddlers with ASD have been discussed; differences in the preschool years may begin to reveal islands of preserved skills in the presence of the social-communication delays already described. Take Fred, for example.

Fred just turned 3 years old. Both Fred and his father have ASD. There are a lot of activities that they enjoy doing together. They watch the same YouTube videos and trailers of movies. Every morning during breakfast they watch a video of an airplane taking off. They watch it at least five or six times, and they have been watching the same video for almost a year. Neither father nor son sees anything wrong with this, although it troubles Fred's mother, who feels that her husband is encouraging Fred to be repetitive. When Fred wants to watch the video again, he moves his father's hand to the mouse so he can reclick the play button. Fred has very little spontaneous spoken language; when asked a question, Fred answers with just one or two words, if he answers at all, or he may simply repeat the question. But he can recite entire scenes of dialogue from his favorite movies, such as *Despicable Me,* which he has repeatedly watched without ever tiring of it.

Echolalia Fred's tendency to repeat what was just said to him is called *immediate echolalia.* Fred's therapist, Sue, is Australian, and when she leaves and is saying good-bye, she will say, "Good-bye, darling." Fred often repeats back, "Good-bye, darling" with Sue's Australian accent. Here are some more examples:

> Adult 1: Fred, what do you want for lunch: pasta or a sandwich?
>
> Fred: Pasta or sandwich, eat sandwich.

> Adult 2: Let's go play in the garden.
>
> Fred: Yes, play in the garden. (runs to the garden)

> Peer at preschool: Look, it's a dinosaur.
>
> Fred: Look, it's a dinosaur. (both children run toward the dinosaur)

Fred's ability to recite long sections of language from movies and television is called *delayed echolalia,* or *scripting.* Although in earlier times therapists tried to extinguish this kind of repetitive speech in children with ASD, most clinicians now believe that echolalia often is used by children with ASD to serve a communicative function—to provide a way to fulfill their conversational turn when they don't know what they should say or don't understand what is being said to them. For example,

Fred is able to recite scripts from his favorite movies and books. When he is upset and is trying to calm himself down, he will use the phrase from *Despicable Me,* "I don't cry, I'm British" (he is not British!).

Therapists often will work with children with echolalia to bridge echoes into more communicative language. Echolalia, particularly the delayed kind, is not something that is seen very often in typical development. Typically developing toddlers may echo as they acquire their first words and sentences, but they get past it fairly quickly, and their echoes are only a little bit ahead of what they can produce on their own. Parents often feel mystified at the length and complexity of the language children with ASD are able to echo, especially in comparison with the limits of their spontaneous speech. Although there is little understanding about how children with ASD accomplish these extended echoes, they do appear to be somewhat disconnected from the language used for communication and don't seem to draw on the same psychological processes.

Some psychologists have argued they represent a particular kind of information processing, called *gestalt* or *holistic,* which people often use to take in visual information, such as looking at an object and reconstructing a picture of the object in your mind. This processing creates a mental image of the whole object or scene without analyzing it into its component parts. It's a valuable way to be able to think and allows us to recognize particular objects or places we've seen before; it's probably also used to recognize faces of people we've met.

Parents often feel mystified at the length and complexity of the language children with ASD are able to echo, especially in comparison with the limits of their spontaneous speech.

A different approach is generally used when listening to and learning language, though. It doesn't take in the whole of what is heard in one chunk, but rather analyzes it word by word or even sound by sound. This kind of sequential processing is typically used for things we hear, at least partly because they come into our brains bit by bit over a span of time, rather than in one simultaneous package as visual information can. Children with echolalia may be more able to make use of gestalt processing for material they hear than the rest of us, and that may account for some of their uncanny echolalic abilities. There is a downside, however; children with echolalia seem less able than their peers to switch to a way of taking in auditory information that allows them to break it down into its component words, syllables, and sounds and use these pieces as building blocks to acquire language. Although therapists may be able to help them learn to do that, the switch between processing styles seems to come less easily to them. This may be one reason why people with autism often report that they are better visual than auditory learners; it may not be that their visual senses are better but rather their preferred style of making sense of information is better suited to things they see than to those they hear.

In any case, two things are important to know about echolalia. First, not every child with autism echoes. Second, children who echo generally have a better chance of acquiring spoken language than those who do not produce any language at all, so it should be seen as a positive sign. SLPs can work with echolalia to teach children how to break their echoed language down into smaller pieces and interchange them and bring changes on them in the service of learning to use a more analytic form of thinking about language as well as acquiring the forms needed to accomplish communication. Children with echolalia, particularly those who use a lot of scripted language, are showing language behaviors that are not part of the typical developmental sequence. Echolalia is one example of the way in which the development of preschoolers with ASD is outside the typical order of development.

Other Characteristics of Language Development in Autism in the Pre-school Years Other characteristics of language development in autism in the preschool years can include using idiosyncratic language or unusual words to convey their meaning. It is also common to observe difficulty with use of pronouns in which the child will use his or her name, such as, "Fred wants ice cream," rather than, "I want an ice cream." The child may also reverse the pronouns *I* and *you,* saying, "You want ice cream," rather than "I want ice cream."

Pretend play blossoms during the preschool years in typical development. Children begin acting out scenes of familiar activities, imitating what they have heard others say and do. They often will use toys or other objects to represent the props in these scenarios, pretending a block is a telephone and putting it up to their ear to "talk to Grandma," for example. Later in the preschool years, children enjoy enacting fantasy events, often involving superheroes, and take roles within the play, which they negotiate cooperatively with peers. Children with ASD show less interest in these kinds of pretend play than their typically developing peers.

> Children with ASD show less interest in these kinds of pretend play than their typically developing peers.

They often prefer to play with objects in ways that involve more concrete motor and sensory exploration. For example, they may prefer to spin the wheels on a car than pretend it is driving to the park.

Specialized interests is another area in which preschoolers with ASD may show unusual development. Some preschoolers with ASD develop an intense interest in numbers and letters; they may know all their letters at a very early age and may even begin to read words. The unusual ability to read during the preschool period is called *hyperlexia* and is present in only about 10% of children with ASD, but it is rarely seen outside of the syndrome. Even children who don't begin reading may have a very high interest in number and letter puzzles and may be able to name or recognize all the letters. This is just one common form of special interest in preschoolers; some may take intense interest in dinosaurs or something more unusual, such as wash-

> The unusual ability to read during the preschool period is called *hyperlexia.*

ing machines. Although typically developing children can show these interests too, they are generally less often seen and less intense. Unlike their typically developing peers, the interests of children with ASD often are an island of apparent skill or expertise among other areas of development that lag behind their peers.

In summary, young children with ASD do not play in the same way as their typically developing peers. Although all preschoolers like repetition and are happy to hear the same book or watch the same video repeatedly, the difference is that children with ASD are often interested in repeated experiences that would not appeal to their typically developing peers. A child with ASD may lie on the floor and watch the wheels of a toy car go around, often for hours if left undisturbed. A typically developing child might enjoy lining up all the toy animals in the house to have a "parade" now and then, but a child with ASD may line up the animals at each opportunity to play with them and be upset if interrupted by another child who wants to join in the play or play another way. Children with ASD are also less likely to show the kind of pretend play that is the hallmark of the preschool period. Although typically developing preschoolers enjoy enacting the roles of family members (e.g., mommy, daddy), people in the community (e.g., doctor, mail carrier), or superheroes and will organize play around these pretend scenarios, children with ASD do not seem inclined to this kind of imaginary activity.

About 25% of children who have ASD develop seizures, often during the preschool period. These can be managed by a physician in the same way they would be for a child who does not have ASD. The reason the appearance of seizures is quite high in children with ASD in comparison with their typically developing peers probably stems from the same reason children have ASD in the first place—differences in the development of their brains and the mechanisms that carry messages from one part of the brain to another lead to both outcomes.

ASD at School Age

Teacher: Sydney, please put your coat away.
Sydney: I don't have a coat. I have a rain jacket.

Sydney attends an inclusive third-grade classroom for students with ASD. She is one of five students with ASD and the only girl. She has made progress over the years and has been receiving therapy services since she was very young. Now that she is getting older, she is finding the social demands both in school and out of school challenging. She doesn't always seem to understand the hidden rules and is quite literal in her understanding of language. Sydney is having a hard time being part of the group and making friends. She tends to say what she thinks and feels and doesn't realize that what she says can hurt other people's feelings. Sydney accidentally bumped her elbow one day in class. Her teacher, who saw it happen, said, "Ouch. It really hurts when you hit your funny bone." Sidney became very upset, "It's not funny. It hurts!" Her teacher tried to explain that it is called a funny bone, but Sydney was too upset to listen. On another occasion, Sydney was in the speech room waiting for the other students to come for their therapy session. She was very upset that the other students were late. Julie the SLP told her, "It's okay, Sydney. They are only a few minutes late. Maybe they finished music late." Sydney looked up at the clock. She was very upset and said, "No, they are 6 minutes and 18 seconds late!"

Language and Cognitive Skills   Nirit Bauminger-Zviely (2014) summarized research on children with ASD in the 6- to 12-year age range. This review revealed that children with ASD show significant growth and change during the school years. Cognitive and language functions show the greatest degree of growth, whereas social and adaptive skills continue to lag behind. For example, although 84% of children with ASD tested at age 2 score below the normal range on intelligence tests, only 40% score below the cutoff for ID by school age. Thirty-eight percent score within or above the average IQ range of 85–115, whereas the rest score in the borderline range, with IQs of 70–84. Similarly, 60% of 2-year-olds diagnosed with ASD show little or no expressive language, but 88% have some functional spoken language by age 9, and 32% can carry on a conversation. The severity of impairments due to autism in the areas of cognitive and language performance tends to decrease during the school years. If your young child is scoring very low on tests of language and cognition, then there is still a good possibility that the situation will improve, especially with intensive, evidence-based intervention during the preschool and early school years.

Social Skills   Social skill impairments, which form core symptoms of ASD, are more persistent. Lack of peer relationships is one of the diagnostic signs of ASD in school-age children. Studies of children with ASD during lunch and recess times find that they show fewer positive responses, more negative responses, and less engagement in play than peers with either typical development or other developmental disabilities, although they show more successful interactions with adults. Children with LFA at school age tend to use positive but simple social initiations, such as standing close to peers or echoing others' words. But they are less likely to initiate play or imitate peers than children at the same IQ level without ASD.

Social skill impairments, which form core symptoms of ASD, are more persistent. Lack of peer relationships is one of the diagnostic signs of ASD in school-age children.

Children with HFA show relatively passive social interactions, including eye contact (but not combined with a smile) and proximity, whereas typically developing peers show a broader and more active set of social behaviors, such as sharing, talking, and helping. Children with ASD also show less spontaneous social interactions and rely on prompting from others to interact. One study (Macintosh & Dissanayake, 2006) of playground behavior of school children with ASD found most time was spent in structured play with rules, solitary play, or just watching others, whereas typically developing peers spent greater amounts of time in spontaneous, imaginative play with others.

Conversational Skills   Conversational skills of school children with HFA show similar difficulties. They are less likely to answer questions, more likely to repeat questions or provide unrelated or bizarre answers, and less able to engage in extended talk with peers than children with other disabilities. They are more likely to engage in monologue speech than back-and-forth conversation and more likely to walk away without closing an interaction.

Friendships   Friendships pose even higher requirements than casual social interactions, and children with both LFA and HFA report fewer friends than typical peers or other children with developmental disorders. Still, one study

(Solish et al., 2010) reported that half the children with ASD did have at least one good friend, and children with friends showed levels of prosocial behavior, such as sharing and smiling, that was similar to those seen in typically developing peers. Although friendships between children with ASD and typically developing peers seem to elicit more complex social behaviors from the child with ASD, friendships between children on the spectrum seem to be more balanced and allow children with ASD the opportunity to take leadership within the friendship, which doesn't seem to happen much in friendships with typically developing peers.

Siblings Siblings also seem to be particularly important social partners for children with ASD. One study (Knott et al., 2007) showed that children with ASD were actively engaged in interaction with their siblings 66% of the time spent together, a level much higher than when they played with nonrelated peers. Siblings seem to play an especially important role in supporting social interactive skills for children with ASD.

Restricted and Repetitive Behaviors Restricted and repetitive behaviors (RRBs), the second major category of symptoms for children with ASD, also undergo changes during the school years. RRBs are generally divided into three types: 1) repetitive sensorimotor behaviors, such as hand and finger mannerisms, spinning, rocking, and peering at objects; 2) insistence on sameness, such as always needing to sit on the same chair, engaging in compulsive rituals, and being unwilling to tolerate the smallest changes in established routines; and 3) special interests, including intense hobbies, preoccupations with odd topics, and strong attachment to unusual objects. Research suggests that younger children and those with LFA are more likely to show sensorimotor RRBs, whereas school-age children and those with HFA are more likely to show insistence on sameness. Still, 39% of school-age children with HFA are reported to show sensorimotor RRBs. Special interests are seen in both groups; nearly 75% of children with ASD are reported by parents to have a special interest, whereas only a third of typically developing children do (Danovich, et al., 2009).

Academic Skills Studies (Heumer & Mann, 2010; Nation et al., 2006) of academic achievement in school-age children with ASD suggest that basic reading and rote memory skills are less impaired than reading comprehension, written expression, handwriting, and problem solving. Students with ASD generally do better on routine tasks, such as multiplication tables, than abstract or conceptual tasks, such as drawing inferences from what they read.

Children with ASD, particularly those with HFA, often show good decoding skills in reading and are able to recognize and sound out words. They have more trouble comprehending the meaning of what they read and have special trouble comprehending fictional stories that rely on understanding characters' goals, plans, and points of view. Many psychologists believe that the reason for these difficulties stems from another cognitive style that seems to be characteristic of children with ASD—weak central coherence. Dr. Uta Frith identified this style in the 1980s, based on the observation that people with ASD often seem to focus on the smallest possible parts of things. They may actually perceive details better than the rest of us but often fail to put the details together into a coherent whole, or they fail to "see the forest for the trees." This may lead readers with ASD to focus on individual words rather than larger meanings, resulting in difficulty making sense of what they read.

Deficits in executive function are a second cognitive area often implicated in the academic difficulties of students with ASD. These are cognitive capacities that allow for goal-directed behaviors such as planning, generating alternative solutions to problems, dealing flexibly with obstacles, and holding things in mind to perform processes such as adding two three-digit numbers in your head. Executive function has been shown to be highly related to success in school for typically developing students, and executive function difficulties have been well documented in students with both LFA and HFA, particularly in the areas of planning and flexibility. It is thought that these difficulties contribute to the problems students with ASD experience in achieving their potential in school.

> Executive function difficulties have been well documented in students with both LFA and HFA, particularly in the areas of planning and flexibility.

ASD in Adolescents and Adults

Gio and Emanuel are adolescents with ASD who have special interests that are different from their typically developing peers. Mr. Sanchez, the SLP at their school, runs a social-communication group for five eighth-grade students with the school social worker. Mr. Sanchez is helping the boys share their special interests as a way to support the development of their friendships. Being part of a group and making connections with their typically developing peers are challenges the boys are having. Mr. Sanchez is playing a game called WhoNu to support their social-communication skills. Each player chooses the card for an item he or she likes and doesn't show it to the other players. The cards are then placed in a bag and the players take turns pulling out a card and guessing who the card belongs to. Gio picks out a card with My Little Pony. Two of the boys laugh, "My Little Pony is for girls!" "It's not for girls," said Emanuel, looking down and slightly embarrassed. "I'm a Brony." "What's a Brony? I have never heard of that before," said Mr. Sanchez. "You know, it's when you're a boy and you like My Little Pony." "No, I don't know," said Mr. Sanchez. The boys showed him a video about Bronies on YouTube.

Mr. Sanchez was taken aback and even more surprised when he found out that three of his five eighth-grade students who attend his speech-language therapy group were all "Bronies," that is, My Little Pony fans, and that this is a growing interest among students with ASD. He also discovered that they had been able to make social connections through their shared interest and they had connected with other "Bronies." Gio then added, "I told my dad that I'm a Brony. At first I thought he would be mad, but the animation is really cool and there is a convention next month. We are going."

Koegel, Koegel, Miller, and Detar (2014) summarized research that tells us that most children with ASD will continue to show improvement in symptoms and in adaptive behavior throughout adolescence, particularly if appropriate interventions and supports are provided. Still, few really outgrow their condition, and continued improvement in young adulthood, although present, is slower.

Entering secondary school is a big transition for many children, and it also presents challenges for students with ASD. These challenges often arise from more complex assignments, more transitions from class to class, less predictability of routines, demands for more independent work and organizational ability, and the need to use abstract and inferential reasoning. Social interactions are more challenging at this age too, with relationships based more heavily on verbal agility and repartee and less on just doing things together. Subtle social cues, a lot of sarcasm, and other nonliteral uses of language come into play, and teasing or bullying can occur. These issues are most likely to affect children with HFA, who will function primarily in regular classrooms and may be expected to keep up with their peers not only in academics but also in the fast-paced social whirl of middle and high school interactions.

The individualized transition plan (ITP) is one support provided by the Individuals with Disabilities Education Improvement Act (IDEA) of 2004 (PL 108-446). The ITP is put in place when the student is 14–16 years old and helps the family and educational team plan for what will happen when students either graduate from high school or age out of the educational system on their 22nd birthday. The plan aims to identify goals agreed on by the family, student, and educational team. It is designed to assist the student in acquiring the skills and supports needed to reach the goals of the post-high school years, which may include college, work, and independent living.

One big change in the outlook for students with ASD is an increase in the number of these students attending college. A survey done by Taylor and Seltzer (2011) revealed that 14% of students with ASD attended college,

> Most children with ASD will continue to show improvement in symptoms and in adaptive behavior throughout adolescence, particularly if appropriate interventions and supports are provided. Still, few really outgrow their condition, and continued improvement in young adulthood, although present, is slower.

> The individualized transition plan (ITP) is one support provided by the Individuals with Disabilities Education Improvement Act (IDEA) of 2004 (PL 108-446). The ITP is put in place when the student is 14–16 years old and helps the family and educational team plan for what will happen when the student either graduates from high school or ages out of the educational system on his or her 22nd birthday.

and some estimates place the proportion even higher. The Americans with Disabilities Act (ADA) of 1990 (PL 101-336) requires colleges to accommodate students with disabilities, but the students must identify themselves and seek the accommodations. Many colleges have specialized supportive programs for students with ASD that help them negotiate the challenges of campus life. It is likely that even more services and supports will be available by the time your young child with ASD is ready to consider college.

> The Americans with Disabilities Act (ADA) of 1990 (PL 101-336) requires colleges to accommodate students with disabilities, but the students must identify themselves and seek the accommodations.

People with LFA may not attend college as adults, but research suggests that nearly half the adults with ASD have some kind of employment, nearly half live either independently or in supported housing, and the proportion of adults with ASD living in institutional settings has dropped significantly since the early 2000s (Howlin, Moss, Savage, & Rutter, 2013). These changes are undoubtedly a result of increased awareness, earlier identification and intervention, and enhanced services for people with ASD at least through the school years. It is very likely that these trends will continue to provide increasingly positive outcomes as heightened public awareness of autism as a lifelong disability and understanding the best ways to manage symptoms and support independence continues to expand.

Several books, articles, and movies are available by and about adults with ASD that your family may want to have a look at:

Books:

- *Born on a Blue Day* (Free Press, 2007) by Daniel Tammet

- *Thinking in Pictures: My Life with Autism* (Vintage, 2006) by Temple Grandin

- *Life, Animated* (Kingswell, 2014) by Ron Suskind

Articles:

- "Parallel Play: A Lifetime of Restless Isolation Explained" by Tim Page in the August 20, 2007 *New Yorker* (*http://www.newyorker.com/magazine/2007/08/20/parallel-play*)

- "Autism's First Child" by John Donvan and Caren Zucker in the October 2010 *Atlantic Magazine* (http://www.theatlantic.com/magazine/archive/2010/10/autisms-first-child/308227/)

Movies:

- *Temple Grandin* starring Claire Danes

- AutismSpeaks provides a list of additional movies about people with ASD and their families at http://www.autismspeaks.org/family-services/resource-library/films-and-documentaries

Although it is natural to think about what your young child will be like as an adult, what is most important during the early years is to focus on understanding the way your child is now and setting in place the most appropriate educational and therapeutic program possible. To help you understand some of the atypical patterns of social interaction and communication you may be seeing in your young child with ASD, we will try to answer some of the questions parents have most often asked us about these issues and give you the best answers we can, in light of our limited knowledge about the underlying causes of social-communication impairments in these children.

Although it is natural to think about what your young child will be like as an adult, what is most important during the early years is to focus on understanding your child as he or she is now and setting in place the most appropriate educational and therapeutic program possible.

What's the Difference Between Talking and Communicating, and Why Does It Matter?

The words *talk* and *communicate* are used to mean pretty much the same thing in most situations. There are some technical differences, though. These are illustrated in Figure 2.1.

Communication is the term with the broadest meaning and refers to any way of getting a message between a sender and a receiver. People communicate, of course, but so do animals; bees communicate to each other about where they found pollen by dancing in patterns that indicate the direction and distance of

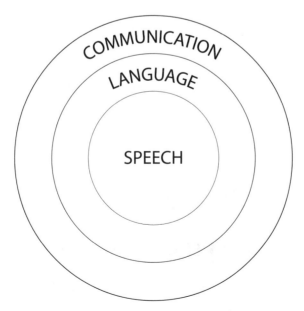

Figure 2.1. Relations among communication, language, and speech.

the find to other bees. Even plants are thought to communicate. For example, sugar maples appear to "warn" each other about insect attacks; bug-free trees near trees that are infested have been seen to send out bug-repelling chemicals to ward off attacks on neighboring trees.

People communicate in a lot of different ways. Messages are sent and received by talking, but we also communicate with gestures (holding out your thumb on a roadway communicates you'd like a ride), what we wear (police wear uniforms to communicate to others what their job is), with facial expressions (smiling when you say, "Shut up!" conveys a different meaning than saying the words without a smile) and a variety of other signals.

Language is one kind of communication; the kind that uses rules to tell us how to combine elements to express different meanings. Language, like communication, consists of several components (see Figure 2.2). *Language form* refers to the rules that tell us how to put sounds, words, and sentences together to express our ideas. Some of these rules are for grammar or *syntax*. They dictate what order words need to go in to enable ideas to be expressed. For example, if we want to identify a bereaved woman as a criminal, we would say, "The widow robbed the bank." But if we want to say that a financial institution took advantage of an elderly lady, then we would need to say, "The bank robbed the widow." Other rules of language form tell how to add parts to words to modify their meanings. For example, these *morphological rules* distinguish between actions that are ongoing (jumping = *jump* + *ing*) and those that are finished (jumped = *jump* + *ed*).

Language form rules also tell how to pronounce different sounds in different situations. For example, when a plural ending is added to the word *cat*

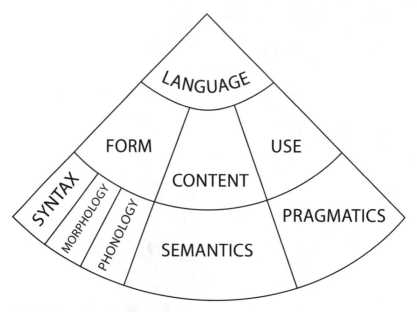

Figure 2.2. The components of language.

in order to talk about more than one of them, the plural in *cats* is pronounced as an /s/. Yet when a plural ending is added to the word *dog,* it is pronounced as a /z/. You may not have realized this before, but if you think about common words and adding plural endings to them, you will see that you automatically pronounce some with an /s/ at the end and some with a /z/. There are rule-based reasons for this, having to do with what kind of sound is at the end of the base word and adding endings that match features of the word's last sound. You probably never knew you knew these rules, but you do, or you wouldn't pronounce *dogs* and *cats* correctly without even thinking about it. All these rules that come under the heading of language form are things that you know without necessarily knowing that you know them and you can use without thinking. This automatic adherence to formal rules is part of what is meant when we say we know a language. These kinds of rules are generally learned more slowly by children with ASD but in more or less the same sequence as other children.

Language content refers to the way in which the meaning carried in words and sentences is understood. For example, when a newly acquainted adult asks a 4-year-old, "Are you married?" we know that he is teasing because the meaning of the word *married* in our culture contains the requirement of adulthood; simply knowing the full meaning of marriage lets us in on the joke. This kind of knowledge is called *semantics* and often is something we know implicitly without being fully aware of knowing it. Children with ASD learn word meanings and can often have large vocabularies. They may use words in a very concrete way, though, and have difficulty understanding that words can sometimes mean more than one thing (e.g., *run* can mean going fast, but it can also mean trying for political office). They sometimes use words in idiosyncratic, private ways as well, and they have difficulty understanding the humor in puns and other word play.

Pragmatics is an additional component of language and the one universally impaired in ASD. Pragmatic rules dictate how words and sentences are used differently in different situations to accomplish social goals. These rules tell that if we want to avoid antagonizing people we don't know very well or who have higher social status, we should say something such as, "Do you think it's a bit chilly in here?" rather than what we really mean, "Close that window!"

Pragmatic rules also provide distinction between sentence meaning and speaker meaning. In other words, people don't always mean exactly what they say. We often use figurative forms of language, that aren't meant to be understood literally. When we ask a stranger, "Would you be kind enough to tell me the time?" we aren't really questioning her level of compassion. We just want her to tell us what time it is, but pragmatic rules dictate that we make requests to strangers in a polite way. When Fred (from the earlier vignette) hears his grandmother call him "sunshine," Fred often responds by saying, "I'm not sunshine. I'm Fred," showing that he fails to understand the figurative use of language.

Many pragmatic rules are never explicitly explained to a growing child, and these social do's and don'ts are constant stumbling blocks for children with

ASD. For example, it is an unspoken rule that if someone gives us a gift we don't like, we tell them thank you and accept it. We don't say we don't like it because that may hurt the person's feelings. For children with ASD, though, therapy and direct instruction may be necessary to teach these unspoken rules.

Language is a peculiarly human form of communication, unlike most of the communication we see in the rest of nature. Its rules allow people to convey an unending number of thoughts, some of which may never have been said before. Although each human language is unique and uniquely connected to the culture in which it's used, all human languages share this property of creativity and the rich complexity of expression it makes possible.

Speech, on the other hand, is a particular mode of language; it's oral expression. Language can be conveyed in a variety of ways—through writing, through formalized gesture systems such as American Sign Language (ASL), or through mathematical symbols in computer languages. *Speech* is a small part of this large set of possibilities; it's the production of sounds with our lips, tongue, teeth, and so forth that make up what we informally call *talking.* You can see that a lot goes into being able to talk. Ideas needs to be created to send to others; different rules need to be learned for putting those ideas into sounds, words, and sentences; and choices need to be made about the right way to say what we mean for each particular social situation. It's pretty amazing that most children do most of this pretty well by the time they are 3 or 4 years old!

Why Isn't My Child with ASD Talking? It shouldn't be too surprising that children with ASD don't usually talk at a young age; what's really surprising is that other children do, given the depth of knowledge involved in producing and understanding speech. A slightly different question needs to be asked to understand why children with ASD are so often delayed in learning language.

What Does It Take to Learn to Talk and Understand Language?

Children are learning a lot about language from their environment and interactions before they start to talk. From the first days of life, infants show preferences for looking at faces and listening to human voices, and these preferences guide them to pay attention to people in their environment. The preferences are general at first; infants will show preference for just about any face (even a smiley face emoticon) or voice. But they begin discriminating around 6 months old and prefer familiar, human faces and voices that are speaking the language to which they are most often exposed. Learning to talk starts at this early stage when children are paying attention to the important visual and auditory signals around them that carry the social information.

There isn't a lot of information about symptoms of autism before the end of the first year, but some studies are beginning to hint that infants who go on to develop autism may start subtly to diverge from typical preference patterns toward the middle of the first year of life (Jones & Klin, 2013). Other studies showed that children with ASD do not look at the face as a whole but are more interested in isolated features and geometric shapes (Pierce, Conant, Hazin, Stoner & Desmond, 2011). Moreover, preferences do not seem to 'tune' to the most relevant signals over the next months of development (Paul, Chawarska, Fowler, Cicchetti, & Volkmar, 2007). In other words, infants who grow into autism may be less interested in faces and voices—particularly the most important faces and voices in their environment—than other infants. Less interest means less attention to these signals, and less attention means less learning. This may be part of the reason language is delayed in children with ASD and why reduced responses to their name and other language input are seen. If a child isn't listening much to language, then learning to produce it is also going to be delayed.

Another reason that children with ASD are slow to begin talking is that language is essentially a refined form of communication. To learn it, the motivation to communicate has to come first; if there isn't a strong need to send messages to others, then there is less drive to learn language as a means to this end. Infants typically begin expressing intentions to communicate at about 8–12 months of age, first with gestures (reaching and pointing), some sounds (babbling), and gaze (looking at others, then looking at what they want to call attention to). Typically developing infants do this for a few different reasons—to get things and to focus adults' attention on things that interest them. This desire to share interest in the world with others is called *joint attention,* and it is a very important part of learning to talk. When we talk, a bit of what we do is make requests, but the larger portion of communication is used to find a topic of shared interest and take turns making comments by adding new information to that topic. Conversation is essentially a cooperative exchange of information about a shared topic. Although these exchanges take place through the medium of sounds, words, and sentences, joint attention lays the basis for the kinds of exchanges infants eventually learn to accomplish with language.

Joint attention lays the basis for the kinds of exchanges infants eventually learn to accomplish with language.

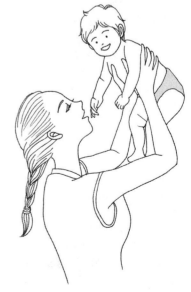

A lot of research has looked at the pre-speech communicative behaviors of children with ASD, and it is quite consistent in showing two important differences between them and other children. First, children who go on to be diagnosed with autism do communicate, but almost exclusively to make requests. They show very few joint attention behaviors, such as looking at what others point to, pointing at things that intrigue them just to share attention with others, or making sounds to get people's attention for its own sake. Although they are showing a basic understanding of what communication is about, they are missing an important aspect of it that supports language development; that is, the ability to establish a shared focus of interest that will eventually serve as a topic of conversation.

The second difference shows up in the way they make requests. Children with ASD tend to do so with sounds or gestures singly. For example, they don't coordinate sounds, gestures, and gaze by pointing at something, making a sound, and looking at a person to get the person to share their focus. Instead, they may just take an adult's hand and move it toward an object they want without looking at the adult, or make sounds without directing their gaze to another person.

If children with ASD can figure out how to make requests, then why can't they do what other children at the same developmental level do and engage in joint attention? Why don't they put sounds, gestures, and gaze together to send a message? Although there are no sure answers, there are a few ways to think about these behaviors that might help us understand. Bloom (1993) argued that what drives children to develop language is their desire to share thoughts and feelings with others that cannot be so easily expressed with the prespeech communication skills they acquire toward the end of their first year of life. Gestures, nonspecific vocalization, and gaze may be adequate to request concrete things. If children want to share what is going on in their minds, though, they need a more precise tool for communication. Bloom argued that it is children's craving for *intersubjectivity,* the ability to let others share in their internal, subjective experiences, that leads them to seek out language forms. Because the core symptom of ASD is a reduced drive for connection with others, it is possible that this reduction in motivation results in less need for the specific means of expression that language provides. This may be another reason children with ASD are slower to learn language than their typically developing peers, even when they have adequate cognitive skills.

Another reason for the differences in communication may lie in the underlying brain differences that have been found in children with ASD. Research shows that some parts of the brain are less interconnected in people with ASD than they are in other people (e.g., Boersma et al., 2012). These disrupted connections among disparate parts of the brain may make sending information from one part of the brain to another difficult. Information usually comes into a part of the brain specialized to deal with input from a particular sense modality (e.g., touch, smell, vision), but the information is usually passed on to other parts of the brain that recognize the information (e.g., that smell is a rose), relate it to things already known and experienced (e.g., I had a rose corsage at my senior prom), and help make decisions about feeling and reacting to the information (e.g., I'm allergic to roses; I need to move away). The disrupted connections in ASD could lead to problems in integrating information from the various senses, recognition, and memory centers, which in turn could lead to difficulty in developing behaviors, such as coordinated looking and vocalizing, that draw on integration of sensations, memories, and intentions. There is a lot of evidence that some of the long-range connections in the brains of children with ASD are not as developed as those in other people (e.g., Uddin, Supekar, & Menon, 2013). This seems like a reasonable part of the explanation for the lack of coordination of looking, gestures, and vocalizing that is often seen in these children.

So, to get back to the original question: What does it take to talk and understand language? The short answer is, it takes a lot.

- It takes experience in infancy paying attention to people talking and watching their faces as they do.

- It takes the ability to identify what others are attending to and share focus on the subject of their interest.

- It takes a strong desire to communicate with others, not only to get things but to share thoughts and feelings.

- It takes a brain that has developed connections between areas that take in information, areas that make sense of the information, and areas that work together to produce a meaningful behavior in response.

- It takes the ability to break phrases down in word-size pieces so they can be recombined into new sentences.

- It also takes some other things not mentioned, such as the motor skills to form the sounds of speech and the cognitive skills to understand words as symbols that stand for objects in the real world.

Missing any of these components can lead to difficulty learning to talk, and children with ASD may be missing several of them.

Why Is My Child Talking but Not Communicating?

Once children with ASD begin talking, it may still be hard to communicate with them. Understanding the difference between two aspects of language, *comprehension* and *expression,* will help us to understand why this is can be true.

Language comprehension refers to the ability to understand what others say. It's obviously different from hearing; an English speaker might hear a news report in Spanish on the radio, but not comprehend its meaning. It's also different from listening, because someone might intently listen to the news report in a foreign language but still not comprehend it. Comprehension goes by a lot of names, including *reception* or *receptive language* and *understanding.* Any of these terms can be used to describe the process that goes on inside the mind of someone who receives language input and draws meaning from it.

Comprehension is a private event; it takes place inside someone's head. We can comprehend language without doing anything about it. For example, students often sit in class listening to a lecture, comprehending the material but not doing anything visible about it until the exam several weeks later. Because of the private nature of comprehension, artificial strategies are needed to find out whether it's happened. That's why your child might be given a language comprehension test that involves pointing to pictures ("Where's the turtle?"), manipulating objects ("Make the horse push the cow") or answering questions ("Is this green?"). If there is not some outward indication that comprehension has happened, then it is hard to tell whether language input was understood.

Language expression, however, means producing words and sentences. Usually it means speech or talking, but writing, ASL, or picture symbols can also be used to express language. You are an important informant to your child's team about how much expressive language your child has. Even though language production is "public," children are often unreliable about producing it on demand. If your child doesn't talk a lot, or prefers only to talk to familiar people, then it may be hard for the educational team to get an accurate idea of what expressive language skills are present, and they may rely on your knowledge. You may be asked to fill out checklists and questionnaires about what your child says so that your team gets the fullest possible picture of your child's expressive skills.

Talking requires a whole range of abilities, as we've seen, and comprehension requires many of the same ones. Although it doesn't require the motor skills needed to produce speech, some additional skills are needed to comprehend language. For one thing, you have to listen. Children with ASD are less "tuned in" to speech, and their attention is less drawn by it than other children, which results in reduced experience with language that can be part of the reason why both comprehension and production are delayed. Although *hearing* is something that just happens when sounds come into our ears, *listening* is an active process that requires focusing on an auditory signal and marshaling attention to make sense of the sounds themselves and their relationship to other things going on, such as what the speaker is looking at. Comprehension requires this kind of focused listening, especially in the beginning stages of language learning.

One reason that children with ASD can sometimes use speech in an unusual or noncommunicative way may have to do with this distinction between expressive and receptive language. If you ask your child with ASD a question or call his or her name, then you may not get an answer. Even after children have learned to use some speech, they may not use it to respond when spoken to. This is likely to be not so much a failure of speech as a failure of listening. Speech is simply less compelling to children with ASD than it is to other children. To get your child to use language to respond to you, you first have to get him or her to listen to what you say. Here are some strategies you might consider using if you are having trouble communicating with a child who doesn't speak when spoken to:

- Instead of calling from across the room, get close to your child when you want to talk with him or her.

- Put your face close up and get him or her to stop paying attention to other things and pay attention to you instead.

- Reward attention to your face and/or voice whenever you get it, and be lavish with tickles, hugs, songs, or anything your child likes when he or she listens to you.

- Make talking with you fun and interesting by including items and activities your child likes when you try to talk with him or her. For example, if you're calling him or her to come in for dinner, after getting up close, getting his or her attention and telling him or her, "Time for dinner," have a little bit of a favorite food in hand to give him or her, or sing, "The food on the table is all read-y, all read-y, all read-y . . ." to the tune of "Wheels on the Bus" when he or she responds with "Okay" or starts coming toward the table.

We've talked about how echolalia is one of the unusual communication behaviors that we see in ASD. We mentioned that echolalia is often used to serve a communicative function. Children with ASD may not know what they should say, even when they begin to talk, because of their difficulties with receptive language. They may have limited understanding of the language they hear, as well as limitations in their ability to turn their thoughts into words and sentences. But they may want to hold up their end of the conversation, at least to some degree. Echolalia is one strategy for doing this, which is why a child may immediately echo back what you just said, or some part of it, when you talk to him or her. For example, if you ask, "Do you want to sit on my lap?" the child might answer, "Sit on my lap," meaning, "Yes, I do."

This kind of answer, by the way, includes what is often called *pronoun reversal*, but this is a misnomer. In fact, children with ASD are *not* reversing pronouns properly. When you ask, "Do you want to sit on my lap?" *my* refers to the person speaking, not a specific person; *you* refers to the person addressed. The appropriate way to answer the question is to reverse the pronoun *my* for *your* ("sit on *your* lap") because the speaker of the answer is no longer the person with the available ("my") lap; it's now the speaker who was invited onto the lap of the previous speaker, who is now the addressee ("you"). *Deictic* (pronounced *day-ic-tic*) refers to these terms whose meaning changes depending on the point of view of the speaker. *My* doesn't mean anyone in particular; it means whoever is talking at the moment; *you* means whoever the speaker is talking to.

There are several pairs of deictic terms: *I/you, my/your, we/they, ours/theirs,* and *here* (near the speaker)/*there* (at a distance from the speaker). Children with ASD often don't understand this deictic function because understanding it involves some degree of taking another person's point of view and that is hard for them. Even typically developing children have some trouble learning deictic terms, although most of the simple pronouns used as examples here are mastered by age 3 in typical development. In any case, when a child with ASD answers, "Do you want to sit on my lap?" with "Sit on my lap," he or she is echoing what was heard and not really reversing anything. So what is often called 'pronoun reversal' is really a form of echolalia.

Another kind of echolalia can also cause communication problems. You may hear your child repeat snatches of favorite songs, commercials, or videos. Sometimes these delayed echoes are self-directed and not communicative at all. Other times they may be used in an attempt to say something that the child does not have the independent language skills to formulate. For example, if asked, "What do you want for lunch?" a child with ASD may sing the jingle from a commercial for a favorite snack. If you ask a child why he or she took a toy from a peer, then you may hear repeated dialogue from a favorite movie in which a character was angry. Learning to search for the function of these echoed utterances can help you understand your child's communication. Once you decipher the function, you can help your child by translating what was meant into more conventional speech. If the child recites a jingle in answer to a question, then you can respond, "Oh, I see, you want Lunchables! You can tell me that. You can say, 'I want Lunchables.' Try that." In his book, *Life, Animated,* the reporter Ron Susskind described how he and his family used the delayed echolalia produced by his son with autism as a bridge to understanding the boy's inner world. Attempting to interpret delayed echolalia can sometimes provide insight into what your child is thinking and feeling.

Why Did My Child Stop Talking?

As we mentioned in Chapter 1, some young children with ASD appear to start talking and then lose words and phrases during the second year of life. Other children develop social skills, such as pointing and making eye contact, that also seem to decrease or regress during their second year. Many parents find this regression distressing and worry that it signals some disease process that could make the child's condition worse. Research reported in several studies (e.g., Lord, Shulman, & DiLavore, 2004) found that this happens in 20%–40% of children with ASD. These studies also reported that the outcomes of children who show this early regression are no worse than outcomes for children who don't regress. Although it is worrying to see a child appear to lose skills, it is not necessarily a sign that things are going to get worse.

Why does it happen? As with so much about autism, it is not known why regression occurs. Some autism researchers have speculated that early regression is related to the differences in the developing connectivity in the young autistic brain; that is, there may be rather specific parts of the brain that enable some early learning. Even the learning involved in acquiring first words may be taking place in relatively limited brain regions. What happens as children learn more language and social skills is that this somewhat isolated initial learning has to "hook up" to other kinds of knowledge—learning grammatical rules, learning about social uses of communication, learning motor coordination to produce longer strings of words, and so forth. If a child has learned some words or some social behaviors such as pointing, but the connections necessary to move on to the next phase of social-communication are not available, then the skills may not blossom into their more widely networked capacities.

Certain brain functions may be carefully timed to coincide with and support these connections. For example, the transition from first words to word combinations usually happens at about 18 months when children are saying about 50 words. The grammatical learning that needs to begin at this time may be "set" to work with a vocabulary of about 50 words, and if the vocabulary is not large enough at the time that this connection is ready to be made, then the "trigger" to get grammar going may not be tripped. If it is not, then the words learned may be shut off from the other brain processes that would normally integrate them with grammar, meaning, and motor skills. Without the pathways that guide the skills to be integrated into higher levels of social cognition, the initial skills may be stuck in a form that becomes isolated from function and may simply wither away.

This is a matter of speculation. Parents who observe this kind of regression should certainly seek evaluation for their toddler if they haven't already. But if the child is in an intervention program, then continuing in a high-quality program will be adequate to address the child's needs.

Will My Child Learn to Play?

You may have heard the expression, "Play is the child's work." People say this because play is the medium through which children accomplish a variety of developmental objectives. *Early exploratory play,* which is seen in the first year of life, helps children learn about their body and how it can affect the world. What does this feel like when I touch it? What does this sound like when I squeeze it? What will happen if I push this or pull that? What will happen if I crawl over there? Infants strive to learn about objects through all their senses; they touch things to feel their shape and texture, throw things to see where they go, bang things to hear how they sound, and mouth things to see how they taste. This kind of sensorimotor learning is typical of the first year of life and is necessary for children to learn about the physical world and what their actions can do in it.

Children's play changes around their first birthday. They gradually become less exploratory. Rather than throwing, banging, and mouthing everything they get their hands on, they begin using different objects for different things—using them the way they've seen other people do. If you give your 1-year-old child a brush, then he or she is likely to try to brush your hair with it; if he or she finds a car, then he or she is likely to roll it on its wheels. This change to conventional uses of objects or *functional play* is sign that that child is no longer only interested in learning about the object itself, but also in its social function and is trying to be like the other people and use objects in the same way others do. This change signals the child's dawning recognition that he or she is part of a world not only of physical objects but also of socially shared activities.

Children begin to show another new play behavior around 18 months. They start to pretend. *Pretend play* is a very important milestone for several reasons. First, it is a form of symbolic thinking; children who engage in pretend play let one item, such as a block, stand in for something else, such as a telephone. When they hold a block up to their ear and pretend to talk on it, they are practicing the skill of representational thinking, holding an image in mind as they project the image onto something in the real world and act on it *as if* it were the imagined object. Symbolic or representational thought is the first step toward abstract thinking, which allows for all our human achievement and creativity. Being able to hold an idea in mind and do something about the idea in the real world is the first step in this direction. That's one reason why play is such an important part of a child's development; it provides the opportunity to practice symbolic thinking and begin to move on to more complex kinds of representational thought.

Pretend play also is important for social development. Children who pretend together learn to use their symbolic thought processes in cooperation with others to create shared scenarios and engage in intersubjectivity as a driving force for learning language. The only way to share things they imagine is to tell others about them, so pretend play can serve as an engine of language development. Children learn other social skills through pretend play, such as taking another person's role and seeing how it feels to walk in their shoes ("I'll be the mommy; No, don't break your toys, baby!"), how to organize a sequence of actions to accomplish a goal ("Let's play school. I'll be the bus driver and you can ride the bus to school, then we'll get off the bus and play in the playground. When the bell rings we'll go into school and you be the teacher"), and how to negotiate and compromise ("I want to be the doctor, too, so let's take turns; first you be the patient, then we'll switch").

Infants with ASD often engage in *exploratory sensorimotor play* during their first year of life. In some cases, they may begin to show unusual forms of exploration, such as preferring to smell objects, peering at them intensely, lining objects up, or being fixated on one object. In other cases, their play can look fairly typical in the first year. It is around the first birthday that differences in play are most often noticed in children with ASD. Many do not reduce the amount

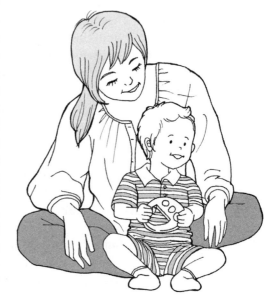

of exploratory play they use. They may make the transition to functional play more slowly than other children. Pretend play can be difficult for children with ASD to achieve. Perhaps play is not at the top of your list of worries about your child's development; but if you think about all the important skills children typically practice while playing, then you can begin to see why play needs to be part of your child's repertoire of activities.

The good news is that if children do not learn to play on their own, they can be taught. Research by Connie Kasari and her colleagues (Kasari, Gulsrud, Freeman, Paparella, & Hellemann, 2012) showed that children with ASD can be taught simple play skills and learning these skills contributes to improved outcomes after several years, particularly in their use of spoken language. Behavioral approaches are sometimes used to teach functional play skills to children with ASD. Research by Kasari and her team suggested that it is important to include more naturalistic approaches that emphasize flexible use of objects, child choice, and pleasurable engagement to get beyond functional play to more pretend-like behavior. Your child's team can help your child make the transition from exploratory play to conventional object use by teaching the child to imitate conventional activities with toys. When functional play is achieved, more truly playful, pretend behaviors can be presented as models to the child in activities of high interest and appeal (see Chapter 7).

Will My Child Learn to Play with Other Children?

Although learning to play in age-appropriate ways with toys is a challenge for many children with ASD, learning to play with friends is even more so. Most children with ASD will need some support from their educational team to develop play skills during their early years, but at some point you will want them to learn to play not only with a supportive adult but also with peers. This kind of support usually comes under the heading of social skills training, and it can begin as soon as the child has some functional play skills and opportunities to interact with peers.

Social skills training will typically occur by about age 3 when the child begins preschool. Teaching strategies for peer play may involve modeling and practicing social-communication skills with an adult therapist. One evidence-based program aims to teach young children to enter a group of peers playing (Beilinson & Olswang, 2003). It has the children learn a simple script. Children are coached to practice the script with a therapist, then they are introduced to a peer play setting and coached by the adult to use the script to enter the play.

Video modeling is another evidence-based approach often used to encourage peer play. Children with ASD are shown a video, either homemade or purchased, that shows children displaying a targeted sequence of behaviors, such as asking a peer to join in a game. The child watches the video with the therapist, discusses what happened, then reenacts the sequence seen on the video with the adult several times. The child is later taken to a group of peers and coached to use the sequence from the video to invite a peer to play a game.

Training peers to support interactions with children with ASD is an additional teaching technique with a strong basis in evidence for teaching social skills to children with ASD. These methods provide simple instructions to typically developing children and structure opportunities for them to interact with peers with disabilities. *Buddy Time* is one program that uses this approach (English, Shafer, Goldstein, & Kaczmarek, 1997). This program is instituted in a typical preschool or kindergarten classroom and takes about 20 minutes

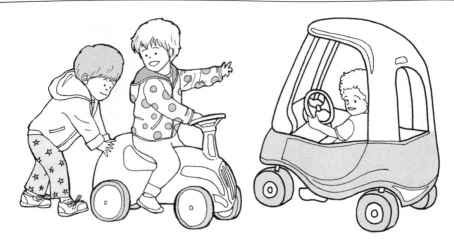

3–5 times per week. Each child is assigned a buddy, and buddies rotate so everyone eventually gets a chance to buddy up with everyone else. The class is taught a series of buddy time rules. At first the rule is simply

• STAY

The buddies must stay together for the entire buddy time period in order to earn a prize. Every buddy pair, both with and without a child with ASD, has a chance to win a prize. This creates an incentive for the typically developing children to keep their buddy with ASD with them, rather than letting the buddy drift off to solitary activity. Once the buddies can stay together, usually after a week or two, a new rule is added:

• STAY

• PLAY

Now to earn a prize, the buddies are required not only to stay together but also to choose a toy or activity and engage with it together throughout the buddy session. After another week or two the final rule is added:

• STAY

• PLAY

• TALK

Here is where the bulk of the peer training happens. Peers are instructed to say their buddy's name, talk about the play, respond to something the buddy says or does, repeat it, then say more about it, ask their buddy a question, and so forth. The peers practice buddy talk in their large classroom group before breaking off into pairs to stay, play, and talk together. Research using this program showed that it increased peers' overtures to classmates with ASD and that the children with ASD also directed more overtures to their typically developing peers.

These are just a few examples of strategies that have been developed to help young children with ASD enhance their play with peers. Although being

Walk over to your friend.

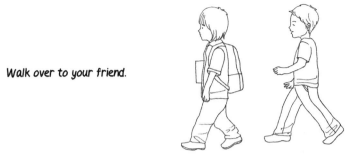

Watch your friend.

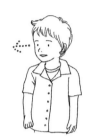

Get a toy like your friend is using.

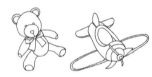

Do the same thing as your friend.

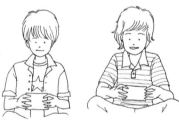

Tell your friend an idea.

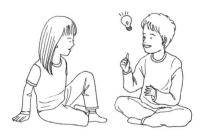

From Beilinson, J., and Olswang, L. (2003). Facilitating peer-group entry in kindergartners with impairments in social communication. *Language, Speech, and Hearing Services in Schools, 34*(2), 157; adapted by permission.

around typically developing children in itself will not teach the necessary play and interaction skills, young children with ASD can learn to develop friendships with encouragement, modeling, coaching, and practice. What's more, their peers can learn to help them. The kinds of prosocial skills that are taught in these programs don't only benefit the child with ASD, then. Typically developing peers can learn empathy and kindness from the opportunity to support a child with a disability. Most parents whose typically developing children are involved in these peer-based programs see benefits for their own child as well.

When children with ASD share an interest with a peer, this can be the basis of their play and the development of their friendships. Parents can encourage their children with ASD to get interested in things that their peers find appealing too, such as popular superheroes and video game characters. Steven Shore (Shore & Grandin, 2003), an adult with ASD, described the importance of developing sharable interests in children who have ASD when they are very young in order to have links to peers. Here's how this worked for Fred's family.

Fred's parents were eager to teach Fred how to play with other children. He started part time at a preschool 3 days per week but did not know how to interact with the other children. Fred's parents didn't want him to miss out on being around other children and playing with them, despite his limited interest in peers.

Fred explored a variety of play materials when given the opportunity to play with peers, but he needed prompts from the adult to move from one activity to the next. He enjoyed playing with the sand, chalkboard, climbing frame, and balls. He sat with the other children during block and sand play and played in parallel with them. He observed the other children and when there were fewer children around, he initiated play with them nonverbally. He was more verbal in a one-to-one setting with an adult.

The SLP helped Fred's parents plan short playdates, visits to the local library for read-and-sing activities, and visits to the local park. Their initial goal was for Fred to play alongside his peers and stay with the small group. They knew that if they could get him into the library and he heard his favorite songs being sung, then he would sit and attempt to sing along. But getting him into the library was a challenge. They were advised by their SLP to build gradually. First, they simply entered the library while he was in his stroller and quickly left. Later, they were able to stay for a few minutes, look through one of his favorite books, and play with playdough. After several trial runs, they were able to attend a story hour with the other young children. Fred sat with the other children and imitated the actions for a song he knew well. He didn't interact with the other children, but he became aware of their presence and started to watch what they were doing, showing an interest in them. This was his first step toward play with other children.

In addition, playdates were organized with Oscar, the son of family friends, in parallel to the library visits. Oscar was a year younger than Fred and proved to be a well-matched playmate. The playdates were initially short, lasting for about 45 minutes. Both Fred and Oscar loved penguins and dinosaurs; this shared interest between the boys was the starting point. They visited the local zoo and enjoyed looking together at the penguins. At first there were no true verbal exchanges. Oscar would make comments and would ask questions, but Fred didn't respond, although he would hold Oscar's hand. They would comment on what they saw but not to each other.

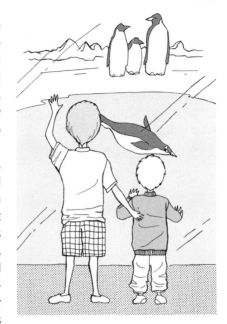

After a few weekly short visits to the zoo, Fred and Oscar independently held hands, and Fred announced, "Go see penguins." They ran to the penguins on their own and had their first verbal exchange when Fred answered Oscar's question about Fred's favorite penguin, saying, "The big one." Their playdates were expanded and later they started to visit the Natural History museum to see the dinosaurs. It was their shared interests in penguins and dinosaurs that helped their friendship to flourish.

It is a good idea for parents to encourage structured play when setting play-dates for their children with ASD. Nonverbal games such as freeze tag are excellent choices. Modified games such as musical chairs or "Duck, Duck, Goose" can be used to encourage participation for the child with ASD in a way that is fun for the playmate as well. Musical chairs can be played so that the children do different actions when they hear the music and when it stops they sit down but no chairs are removed. They could pretend to walk like elephants taking large steps, walk tall like giraffes reaching their arms up, or take tiny, quiet steps like mice. Changing the rules of the games can also be useful for the child with ASD as it addresses challenges with flexibility and at the same time makes the game interesting for the playmate. Board games such as Candy Land can be played with modified rules (e.g., they eat the candy first and then they have to do an action to 'work off the candy'). Simple cause and effect games can be played so that the children need to reference each other nonverbally (e.g., rolling or throwing a ball to a partner only when the partner looks at the peer).

CONCLUSION

This chapter explained some of the common features of ASD and how they relate to typical development. But in all this talk of differences, it's important to remember the ways in which your child with ASD is just like every other child. Like all children, those with ASD need adults to direct their attention to the important things, keep them safe, and help them learn how to get along with others. All children need the opportunity to explore, make mistakes, and get into trouble and experience the consequences. All children need to interact with peers, get dirty, discover things that are fun for them, and learn ways to enjoy other people. Most of all, all children need their parents' love, support, and approval. Although children with ASD may need some extra help that other children don't, they will still need all the things that other children do. Don't forget those things as you work with your educational team to create a therapeutic program for your child.

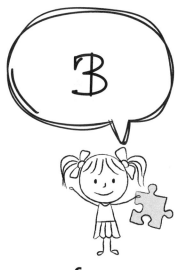

What Are the Social Communication Symptoms of Autism Spectrum Disorder, and How Are They Evaluated and Treated?

We've talked a great deal about the typical course of development of many of the characteristics that serve as signs of autism, and what goes into diagnosing children with ASD. Two major classes of symptoms have been identified: 1) social communication and 2) restrictive, repetitive patterns of interest and behavior. Although both types of symptoms need to be present in order to make a diagnosis, this chapter focuses on the first set of symptoms, those that have to do with social-communication, interaction, and language, because these are the symptoms that will generally receive the most effort on the part of your intervention team, the symptoms you will be most involved in addressing, and the ones that can be coaxed into helping the child achieve the best level of function. Let's first review what these social communication symptoms look like in young children.

WHAT WILL THE TEAM LOOK FOR WHEN EVALUATING A CHILD?

An educational team will look for two things in an assessment for a child suspected of ASD. First, they will look for the level of development a child is showing, relative to age, in the major areas of development such as language, problem-solving, motor, and adaptive skills. They will use a range of standard tests and parent-report instruments to gather this information. Second, they will look for symptoms of ASD: the social-communication and restrictive, repetitive behaviors that are core to the syndrome (see Boxes 3.1 and 3.2). As they did with the developmental measures, the team will gain some of the information from direct testing and observing your child and some from asking you to complete questionnaires or participate in interviews to get a fuller picture of your child's profile.

 Social Symptoms

Social symptoms are nonverbal behaviors that often lead parents to worry about their child's development before the child starts talking. They include

- Reduced tendency to look and smile at others

- Reduced likelihood to imitate others' actions, as in play with toys

- Reduced participation and enjoyment in infant games, such as Peekaboo

- Reduced babbling, especially back-and-forth babbling with others

- Increased and long-lasting use of unusual sounds

- Reduced use of gestures, especially pointing, to get others to pay attention or do something; also reduced ability to follow others' gestures, such as difficulty looking toward where others point

- Reduced interest in other people's talk; delayed response to hearing name

- Reduced interest in sharing things and experiences with others; lack of showing objects

- Reduced ability to follow others' attention to objects (responding to joint attention) or signal others to share attention to an object of interest to the child (initiating joint attention)

- Limited initiation of communication, except to get things or help

- Unusual social initiations, such as licking or smelling others

- Using others as tools by grabbing their hand or arm to take them to something the child wants without looking at their face

- Limited interest in sharing enjoyment with others by looking at them with warm facial expressions or finding pleasure in being with others; limited responses to praise or attention from others

- Failure to learn to play with toys as others do, in functional ways (e.g., lining up blocks in a row instead of building a tower)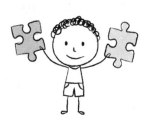

- Failure to develop pretend play (e.g., persisting in exploring objects' shapes and textures rather than pretending the object is something else)

- Preference for solitary activities; failure to notice other children

Language/Communication Symptoms

Language/communication symptoms are usually noticed when other children begin talking; parents become concerned because the child appears delayed in acquiring speech.

- Delayed acquisition of spoken language; slow to acquire first words and sentences

- Inability to follow simple instructions or respond to name

- Immediate or delayed echolalia

- Unusual rhythm, melody, or intonation in speech

- Echoing pronouns instead of properly reversing them ("Pick you up" instead of "Pick me up") for a long period of time

- Verbal rituals; repeatedly having to say or hear the exact same words the same way

- Speech that sounds too stiff and grown up for the young child, who may sound like a "little professor"

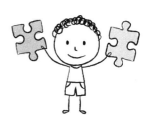

Apart from helping make a diagnosis of ASD, the assessment of social-communication symptoms, especially, helps the team identify where your child is showing strengths in interacting with others, identify targets, and prioritize needs in an intervention program. Let's look at the social-communication assessment in more detail to show how it helps the team to develop an educational plan for a child with ASD.

What Does a Communication Assessment Look Like?

As we've said, there isn't a single, simple test for ASD the way there are IQ tests to identify ID or blood tests to identify diabetes. ASD is identified by observation and history of the symptoms that characterize the disorder. This is made difficult because many of the symptoms of ASD are made up of the absence of or reduction in behaviors that are usually seen, such as the lack of a social smile or a reduced number of attempts to initiate communication. That's why using both direct observation and parent report are so important—to make sure that if a behavior is not seen in a particular assessment session, then its absence is typical of the child and not just an unusual occurrence because the assessment setting is unfamiliar.

There isn't a single, simple test for ASD the way there are IQ tests to identify ID or blood tests to identify diabetes. ASD is identified by observation and history of the symptoms that characterize the disorder.

Setting up situations when the behavior usually would occur and seeing if and how often a child shows it is another way assessment teams try to compensate for the need to show a behavior is not part of the child's repertoire. Barry Prizant, Amy Wetherby, and their colleagues (1997) called this method *communication temptations.* They might, for example, put a treat the child likes inside a big plastic jar with a screw-on lid the child can't open, hand the child the jar, and wait to see whether the child will request help from another person in some way. If so, observers can note not only that the child sought help, but also how the need for help was demonstrated (e.g., speech, gestures, eye contact, a combination of both). Presenting a range of these temptations in an assessment can help the team learn a lot about whether and how a child communicates.

Several assessment instruments that structure these observations are available. The ADOS (Lord et al. 2012) includes a variety of temptations, called *presses* by its authors, to attempt to elicit social-communication behaviors appropriate for children at a range of developmental levels. The Communication and Symbolic Behavior Scales (CSBS-DP; Wetherby & Prizant, 2003), which also involves naturalistic procedures and communication temptations, is another measure often used by SLPs. Instruments like these are designed to find out what a child can and cannot do in terms of social-communication so that strengths can be built on and weaknesses addressed. They also allow a score to be calculated with information across several areas of assessment (e.g., expressive language, receptive language, nonverbal communication). The score can be used to compare the child being assessed with other children who took the test to determine whether the child meets a threshold for autism or shows patterns of scores that differ from what is seen in typically developing children. The ADOS was developed as a diagnostic instrument, so its score is generally compared with a cutoff score that indicates a diagnosis of autism. The CSBS-DP, however, was developed not so much to identify autism as to measure the child's strengths and needs across several areas of social-communication. As such, it is more often used for intervention planning with a child who has already been diagnosed.

So in addition to standardized tests of cognition, language, motor and daily living skills, the assessment of a young child suspected of ASD will usually include an evaluation of strengths and needs in social-communication using a combination of direct observation on a scale designed like the ones just described to tempt the child to display key social-communicative behaviors and information from parents on similar behaviors to make sure that what the team sees in the session is a valid picture of the child's usual behavior.

In addition to standardized tests of cognition, language, and daily living skills, the assessment of a young child suspected of ASD will usually include an evaluation of strengths and needs in social-communication using a combination of direct observation on a scale designed to tempt the child to display key social-communicative behaviors and information from parents on similar behaviors to make sure that what the team sees in the session is a valid picture of the child's usual behavior.

If you have a young child diagnosed with ASD, then you probably went through some months of noticing things about your child's development that were different from what you saw in other children, hoping you were worrying too much and that the child would grow out of it, wondering if you should take the child to see someone, feeling guilty that you hadn't done it sooner, and a whole host of other thoughts and concerns. This is a perfectly natural series of feelings to experience, and many times children do grow out of minor oddities or apparent delays in their first few years. A difference of 6 or 10 months in the age at which a child is diagnosed and begins intervention won't make an enormous difference in long-term outcome. Lilly's story gives us an idea of how this worked in one family.

When Lilly was 14 months old, her parents noticed that although she babbled, she made some funny sounds and often hummed the sounds of her favorite cartoons. She was observed to smile at her parents and grandparents, but she did not seem to be very interested when they would try to get her to imitate them or play games such as Peekaboo. When her parents called her name, she often would not look at them, and they also noticed that she used unusual means of communicating her needs; often pulling the adult's hand to the item she wanted rather than looking at faces and pointing to the object. At about this time, one of Lilly's cousins was diagnosed with ASD at the age of 2½. Lilly's parents began reading about ASD and found out that it tends to run in families. Still, they hesitated to get Lilly assessed. She was so little, what could the testers possibly do? Even if they decided something was wrong, what kind of treatment could there be for a 1-year-old child? They decided to wait and see how things went and hope for the best.

By the time Lilly was 21 months old, all the other toddlers in her playgroup were talking and playing nicely with toys. Lilly still had only two or three words and preferred to be by herself, even during playgroup time. She spent as much time as she was allowed spinning tops or turning toy cars upside down and spinning their wheels around and around as she closely watched them. She did love music, though, and would sit down with the other children when one of the moms led them in a song. Her parents' concern had not lessened, though, seeing her with other children her age, and they decided to schedule her 24-month checkup with her pediatrician early and ask him about her behavior. When they mentioned their concerns, he had them fill out a screening questionnaire for ASD, and they were told that Lilly's score placed her at risk for the disorder. The doctor referred them to a local early assessment agency, and the family reluctantly decided to have Lilly assessed.

Once Lilly's family had their concerns confirmed by means of the screening questionnaire, they were able to gain access to assessment services through the public birth-to-3 system. Let's look at what is likely to happen when they meet Lilly's assessment team.

WHAT TESTS WILL BE USED TO ASSESS MY CHILD?

Part of your child's assessment will consist of tests and measures to determine where in the sequence of development the child is functioning. Since some children with ASD have age-appropriate skills in some areas and not others, the team will want to identify these areas of strength and weakness. There are several kinds of assessment instruments that can be used in this process. We'll describe them for you here.

Standardized Tests

The standardized test is probably most familiar kind of assessment instrument. It is a procedure developed to compare a child's performance with that of other children the same age in order to decide whether the child's performance falls within the normal range. *Normal range* is usually defined as the middle range of scores of children who were part of the test's norming sample, a large group of children, usually at least 100 in each age group, who were given the test as part of its development. The normal range consists of scores that are not the very top scores or the very lowest; usually they are the middle 80%–95% of the scores (it varies a bit from test to test). So, if a child scores in the top 2%–3% of scores, then that score is not considered within the normal range, although it's not usually one to worry about because it is a better score than most children got. Concerns arise for children who score near the bottom of the test's score range, usually the bottom 10%, or sometimes the bottom 2%. Your team may use this kind of score to report your child's performance on a test. If your child got a score at the 9th percentile, for example, then it means that 9% of the children in the norming sample got the same score or lower than your child.

Standardized tests often are used to decide if a child's performance is outside the normal range in a particular area in order to identify a meaningful difference from typical development. IQ tests are one example of standardized tests and are designed to examine the development of a child's cognitive or intellectual abilities—those involved in solving problems (e.g., what to do if you cut yourself), finding and extending patterns, and recognizing similarities and differences. They yield a *quotient* score that reflects how a child does relative to other typical children the same age. Quotient scores are usually measured on a scale in which 100 is the average score for children of a given age, and 96% of children have scores between 70 and

> Standardized tests often are used to decide if a child's performance is outside the normal range in a particular area in order to identify a meaningful difference from typical development.

130. The 70–130 range is usually considered normal for an IQ test. Children who score below 70 (below the 2nd percentile) are considered significantly below the norm in intellectual functioning. IQ tests are used for a variety of purposes, but one is to help identify children with significant ID, formerly called *mental*

retardation. Because they also identify children who score significantly higher than normal (e.g., above 130), IQ tests are also used as part of the identification process for children who are gifted.

IQ tests used to assess children with autism and other disabilities often have several different scales. The most common types are scales that separate verbal abilities (e.g., being able to say and understand words and verbally presented material) from nonverbal (e.g., the ability to recognize and interpret visual patterns without naming or describing them). A motor scale is often included in these tests for very young children because so much early development involves learning how to walk, jump, draw, and use utensils. Many children with ASD score much worse in verbal areas than they do on nonverbal or motor scales. These differences can be a good sign because several studies have found that children who do better on nonlanguage testing in the early years tend to have a better prognosis than those who score low on all scales (Eaves & Ho, 2004). It is important to remember that most standardized tests of this kind are not considered stable until a child is 4 or 5 years old. That means that if children are tested at 2 or 3 years old, as children undergoing assessment for ASD often are, then their scores are likely to change over the next several years. A low score on a test of intellectual ability in the early years does not necessarily mean the score will always be that low. But it does mean that the child is delayed in the tested area *now*, and it is important to provide the child with help to learn the skills that are lagging.

In addition to IQ tests, tests of language function often are used in developmental assessments of children with ASD. Although IQ tests may contain verbal scales, these scales give only a general picture of the level of a child's use of language in comparison with typically developing children. More detailed information often is needed in order to develop an intervention program that builds on the child's current strengths and addresses weaknesses. For this reason, children are often given a standardized language test, such as the Peabody Picture Vocabulary Test (PPVT) or the Preschool Language Scale (PLS), as part of an assessment for ASD. These tests help the team to find out whether the child understands more than he or she is saying, whether he or she knows quite a few words but is not putting them together to form sentences, and what kind of errors the child makes in pronouncing words, forming grammatical sentences, or choosing words to express ideas. Scores from language tests typically are used to establish the child's current (baseline) level of language function, to compare this with functioning after some intervention has taken place, and to pinpoint the areas where the child is ready to learn new language skills that can be addressed in a therapy program.

Scores on standardized tests can be useful for the reasons discussed. They don't diagnose ASD, though. They assess certain aspects of development, but not the core symptoms of ASD. Instruments specially designed to look for those core symptoms are needed in order to make the diagnosis (See Chapter 2). These measures are not standardized tests because they do not yield a score that is directly compared with the scores of typically developing children. Instead, they often are what is called *criterion-referenced measures,* meaning that they identify certain criteria (e.g., Does the child initiate joint attention? Does the child have repetitive behaviors?) and assess whether the child meets each criterion. The ADOS (Lord et al., 2012) is an example of a criterion-referenced measure.

Criterion-Referenced Tests

Criterion-referenced language measures often are used to assess the communication skills of children who are not yet talking. Some language tests can be used with preverbal children to learn how many words they understand (e.g., the PPVT) or whether they can follow simple instructions (e.g., PLS). Criterion-referenced measures are more useful, however, to find out how often (frequency), for what reason (function), and how (form) a child accomplishes communica-

Criterion-referenced language measures are often used to assess the communication skills of children who are not yet talking.

tion. For example, the rate of communicative actions exhibited by a child suspected with ASD can be observed and compared with those seen in typically developing children under the same conditions.

Many tasks on criterion-referenced measures for this purpose involve temptations. For example, an attractive toy may be shown, then hidden, and the clinician tempts the child to ask for it. A child may be offered a bag of toys and invited to pull one from the bag in order to observe whether he or she will share the toy or initiate joint attention to it with the adults in the room. When children are not yet talking, assessors look for other means of communication. Some may be adaptive, such as using a gesture to request a hidden toy, making a sound to call an adult's attention to a toy, or looking at the adult for help with a closed jar. Sometimes, though, children will use less adaptive ways to communicate their needs. A little boy may bang his head on the table when he cannot obtain a toy he wants. A little girl may begin turning around in circles when she cannot open a jar. These behaviors also send a message and are considered communicative, but they do so in a maladaptive, unusual way. Still, they are an important part of the assessment because they tell the team how often these kinds of behaviors occur and what thoughts they communicate.

Replacing these maladaptive behaviors with more appropriate ways to communicate is one of the first goals the team may set. The assessment will also show the team what ideas the child is trying to get across with means other than speech, such as gestures, gaze, and sounds. For the communicative acts the child is already expressing with gestures, gaze, and sounds, the team may target early words, signs, or pictures to communicate these ideas in a more mature way. For communicative functions that the child does not yet express at all, or very infrequently, the target may be to get the child to express these ideas nonverbally, with gestures, gaze, and sounds first, before moving on to more symbolic means of expression.

Play Assessment   Play is another area that often is explored with criterion-referenced assessment. Children with ASD often do not play the way other children do, focusing more on exploring objects and using them in repetitive ways (see Chapter 2). Assessments of play for children suspected of ASD usually consist of giving them opportunities to use play with objects that encourage functional use and pretend, observing how the children use the objects, providing a model of functional or pretend use, and observing whether the child follows the adult's example.

This kind of assessment has two purposes. One is simply to see how the child plays and uses toys because children with ASD often use toys in particular, unusual ways. The other is because using objects in play is related to using words to communicate. Researchers have known for years that typically developing children who show more symbolic or pretend play tend to have more spoken language because, as we've discussed, using toys as symbols involves the same mental processes as using a word to stand for an idea. Both pretending and using words involve symbolic thought—the ability to hold a thought in mind and express it out into the world. These two kinds of behavior—pretending and language—usually go together in typical development. But for some children with disabilities, one form of symbolic behavior may be ahead of the other. If this is true for your child, then the assessment team will want to know, because if play skills are ahead of the child's language level, then it suggests the child is more ready to learn language than if both are similarly delayed. Play assessment will not only help the team describe your child's level of function, but will also help to decide if the child is ready to learn a symbolic communication system, such as speech or sign, or needs to spend more time developing play and preverbal communication skills before focusing on symbolic communication. To show you how this assessment information can be used, here are some of the things that happened at Lilly's assessment when she was nearly 2 years old.

Lilly's parents reported she was saying five or six different words and doing a lot of babbling. The team did an ADOS (Lord et al., 2012). They also used a Mullen Scales of Early Learning to assess her verbal, visual (nonverbal), and motor skills. They used the CSBS-DP (Wetherby & Prizant, 2003) to get a closer look at her communication. Lilly's parents had informed the team that Lilly loves bubbles and the Moomins. They put a Moomins book in a clear box to tempt Lilly and see how she would respond. As soon as Lilly saw the box, she shrieked with joy, "Moo-Meens piz!" Lilly also enjoys puzzles, and she completed an inset puzzle soon after she received it. She also likes banging the puzzle pieces together by her ear and spinning them.

The team met with Lilly's parents and reported that the ADOS (Lord et al., 2012) showed Lilly scored within the range seen in children with ASD. The Mullen showed her motor and visual skills were at age level, but her verbal skills were delayed in both expression and comprehension. The CSBS-DP (Wetherby & Prizant, 2003) showed that Lilly was requesting things in almost all the temptation situations presented, using sounds and her few words, but she hardly ever communicated for reasons other than making requests. Her play skills were observed to consist mostly of turning toys over to look closely at their shape or banging them together to hear the sound they made. Even after modeling feeding a stuffed toy with a spoon, Lilly did not show any pretend feeding. The team recommended that she begin intervention and that one of her goals would be to learn more words for making re-

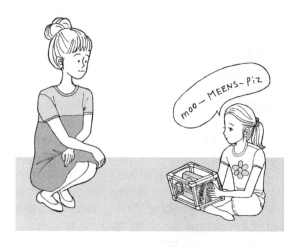

quests; another to use gestures, gaze, and sounds to communicate for joint attention, as well as to work on imitating others and using toys in pretend ways.

WHY WOULD A CHILD WHO IS NOT TALKING NEED TO SEE A SPEECH-LANGUAGE PATHOLOGIST?

Social-communication symptoms are very prominent in diagnosing ASD and are the primary focus of intervention efforts. Many professionals will be involved in this effort, but you may be especially puzzled about the involvement of the SLP if your child is not yet talking. There are two reasons for this. First, the SLP is responsible for doing the criterion-referenced assessment that looks at how your child communicates—how often he or she tries to get ideas across, for what purposes, and in what way. Second, many children who do not talk can be helped by having a symbolic way to communicate that does not use speech and so does not require the high level of motor coordination and imitation skills that are needed for talking. Let's take a look at how this might work.

Juan is a 3-year-old boy who was diagnosed with autism at the age of 28 months. He has been receiving home-based intervention since then. Juan occasionally echoed parts of words after an adult but did not use words to ask for things or interact with others. His mother, Maria, tried very hard to understand his nonverbal ways of communicating, but, more often than not, this resulted in a guessing game that ended in frustration and tears for both. If Juan wanted something and could not reach it himself, then he either pulled an adult by the hand toward what he wanted or he screamed and cried until someone figured out what he was after.

Maria spoke with their SLP to explain how she had repeatedly tried to teach Juan spoken words. For example, when she knew Juan wanted to drink water, she asked him to repeat the word *water,* but he didn't say anything and just became more upset; this often ended with a tantrum. Maria reported that she felt frustrated and sad about the difficulty communicating with her son. The SLP explained that talking can be difficult for children with autism and asking Juan to repeat words at this stage can be frustrating for everyone. Juan may only learn from it that no one can meet his needs unless he screams, and screaming will eventually get him what he wants. The SLP recommended teaching Juan a few signs as a stepping stone toward acquiring verbal language. Although Maria was willing to try this strategy, she's worried— "Aren't signs or gestures only used with children who are deaf? Does deciding to teach Juan signs mean the SLP thinks Juan will never speak? Will using signs discourage him from learning to talk?"

Most children with ASD do develop spoken language, although it may take them until they are 5 or 6 years old. It can be helpful to have an alternative way to communicate that allows the child to express wants and needs during the time when speech is limited. *Augmentative or alternative communication* (AAC) is the term used to describe these methods. Just as there are many ways to get from one place to another (e.g., on foot; by bike, car, train, or plane), there is more than one way for a child to communicate. The team's job is to find the most efficient means of allowing the child to successfully express needs now in order to learn that there is an adaptive way to get messages across. That understanding may be helpful in acquiring speech.

> Most children with ASD do develop spoken language, although it may take them until they are 5 or 6 years old. It can be helpful to have an alternative way to communicate that allows children with ASD to express wants and needs during the time they have very limited speech. *Augmentative or alternative communication (AAC)* is the term used to describe these methods.

It is usually an SLP who evaluates the child's readiness and need for an AAC system, chooses the most appropriate AAC method for the particular child, and teaches the child to use it. AAC systems can be either unaided (e.g., gestures, signs) or aided (e.g., using other tools such as pictures, switches, devices specially designed to reproduce speech, or speech-generating software on consumer electronic platforms, such as iPads).

Many young children who are preverbal start out with signs because signs can easily be modeled, physically prompted, and shaped. Consumer electronic platforms are also quite accessible for young children, however, and also may be helpful. The main point of an AAC system is not what type is used, but that the system provides a more flexible, conventional way to express wants and needs for the child. In this way, AAC can build toward the ability to communicate a wider range of meanings than

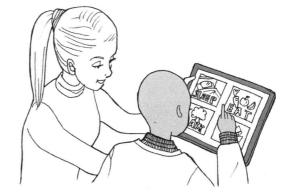

nonsymbolic gestures or vocalizations can achieve. Either speech or an AAC system can help the child take the crucial first step from communication to language. Box 3.3 contains an example of an approach that has been used to teach first signs to preverbal young children with ASD. Let's see how this worked for Juan and his family.

 Five Steps in the SET GO Program for Teaching Signs

S: Select activities and items the child enjoys.

E: Establish a positive rapport.

T: Teach the child to request.

G: Give reasons to use targeted signs by contriving situations.

O: Omit and reduce prompts as child becomes more independent.

Step 1: *Select targeted activities or items.* Create a short list of targeted activities and items the child enjoys. Identify three or four activities and items for which the child will learn the signs.

Step 2: *Establish positive rapport.* Help the child understand that other people can make fun things happen. Engage in activities the child enjoys and find ways to share them. For example, hold the child's hands and sing in rhythm as he or she jumps on a toy trampoline.

Step 3: *Teach how to request using signs.* Use consistent, simple verbal prompt phrases ("What do you want?") as well as physical prompts, and then name the item or action with a sign. For example, provide a closed jar with a treat in it, model the sign for OPEN, physically guide the child to produce the sign OPEN, then open the jar and provide the treat.

Step 4: *Give reasons to sign.* Set up situations in which the child can practice the signs throughout the day; have items from each meal and snack in closed containers so the child must use a sign to request that adults open the container.

Step 5: *Omit or reduce prompts.* Wait before prompting, allowing the child time to produce the sign him- or herself. If he or she doesn't produce the sign, then provide a very small prompt, such as touching his or her hands instead of shaping them fully into the sign for OPEN.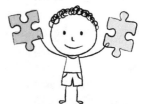

(From Fahim, D. [2011, November]. *Toddlers with autism spectrum disorders: A workshop on intervention strategies and best practices for families and providers.* Workshop conducted at the National Alliance for Drug Endangered Children Conference, Washington, DC.)

Initial attempts to get Juan to use signs to ask for things he wanted resulted in his running away. For example, when presented with a bubble jar, he showed that he wanted bubbles blown for him, but when the SLP demanded he make a sign for BUBBLE, he would look for something else he could get without having to do anything to get it. Maria was concerned, "Is this going to work? He's all over the place and doesn't stay still for a second."

The SLP started off by playing with Juan on the trampoline to establish positive rapport with him. She held his hands, and while he jumped, she simultaneously labeled his action, "Juan's jumping. Jump, Jump, Jump." After 1–2 minutes of jumping, the SLP then started to use sentence completion, "Ready, set . . . ," pausing and waiting for Juan to look at her before she would say "go." The SLP introduced the bubbles after she had Juan's interest. She blew bubbles and simultaneously said and signed BUBBLES in between jumping, which made Juan laugh as he tried catching the bubbles. After doing this a few times, the SLP paused the bubble blowing and said, "Give me five," and then placed her palm out in front of Juan's to give him the opportunity to slap her palm with his palm. As soon as Juan tapped her palm with his hand, she immediately blew the bubbles again.

The SLP showed Maria how to teach Juan the sign for OPEN, which was selected because it can be used for many different requests and situations (e.g., open door, open cookies, open box). Maria held the bubbles in front of Juan and said, "What do you want? Open!" Maria then took Juan's hands, helped him make the sign for OPEN, and then immediately opened the bubble jar and blew bubbles. Because Maria reported that Juan also enjoyed music, the SLP showed her how to prompt Juan to use the sign for MUSIC. Maria first held Juan's hands while he jumped on the trampoline, then, just as the SLP had done, they sat down in between jumping, and Maria gave Juan the musical toy and started to sing a song. Maria then used the same physical and verbal prompts as the SLP. "What do you want? Music!" Juan was willing to allow his mother to help him, and he signed MUSIC.

Together, Maria and the SLP selected four signs representing things Juan most frequently wanted, which included EAT, MUSIC, BUBBLES, and OPEN. The SLP helped Maria think of ways to encourage Juan to use the signs to have his needs met throughout the day. For example, Juan was asked to use the sign for EAT any time he wanted to eat. Juan was asked to use the sign for JUMP whenever he wanted to jump.

Maria and the SLP practiced using the signs for the next 2 weeks. By the end of that time, Juan used the sign for EAT three times, with an imitative prompt and echoed part of the word *ee*. He used the sign for MUSIC with both a partial physical and verbal prompt, and he used the sign for OPEN with a physical and verbal prompt.

Maria told the team, "I was skeptical when the SLP wanted to try signs, but getting him to use them has really helped his behavior. He's calmer and doesn't get upset when he has to wait. He uses the signs for EAT, MUSIC, and sometimes OPEN now. He has also started to make sounds when he signs for EAT. My aunt and his older sister have also learned the signs. Even the man in our local shop has started to sign THANK YOU with Juan."

HOW DO CHILDREN MAKE THE
TRANSITION FROM COMMUNICATION TO LANGUAGE?

Many parents are concerned that if an alternative system, such as signs or computer-generated speech, is introduced, then the child will rely too heavily on the alternative method and never learn to speak. A lot of research looked into this question and generally found that using an alternative system does not seem to keep children from learning to talk. Some studies showed that children who are preverbal who begin using AAC systems have some advantage in acquiring speech (Kasari et al., 2014). It's thought that the AAC system helps children with ASD understand a basic concept about communication that their autism kept them from understanding before—that it is possible to influence others and get what we want by using symbols and sending messages instead of by physically manipulating people. AAC systems seem to help some children with ASD to the "Aha!" moment when they realize, "If I say (or express in some way) something, then others do something. I don't need to drag them by the hand to what I want and hope they get what I need them to do with it. I can use this word/sign/picture to get what I want and they get the message. So that's why everybody has been making those noises with their mouths all this time!" Once this moment is reached, children have a more powerful reason to learn to speak than just doing what others are doing.

An alternative system does not seem to keep children from learning to talk.

Typically developing children seem to have a strong drive to become and act like others around them. That's why their play often involves imitating what others do, and it's one of their motivations for acquiring speech. But part of having ASD is having less motivation in this direction. Learning to talk just to be like others is not a powerful enough reason for children with ASD to go to the trouble of acquiring speech. Acquiring speech is hard! You have to listen carefully to what others say, follow what they look at while they say it to figure out how the words relate to things in the world, chop up the stream of sounds into separate words, create some kind of mental representation or trace of the words to serve as a target for what you want to say, somehow store this memory in your mind so you can find it again when you want it, make very fine motor movements in order to recreate the sounds you've stored in your mind, and adjust those movements minutely to make your sounds match the speech of other speakers in your environment in all the subtle ways that make speech sound right.

Typically developing children seem to have a strong drive to become and act like others around them. That's why their play often involves imitating what others do, and it's one of their motivations for acquiring speech. But part of having ASD is having less motivation in this direction.

If you ever taught baby signs to any of your typically developing children, then you may have noticed that they were able to produce quite a few baby signs before they could talk. That's because the motor skills necessary to form signs with the hands are easier and less precise than the motor skills needed to form the sounds of speech. Of course, you can shape the infant's hands with yours, so the target can be corrected if the child doesn't get it quite right. You may also have seen that knowing baby signs did not stop your infant from learning to talk, and that the signs easily fell away once speech became available. Although the transition may not be quite so natural for children with ASD, there is no evidence that using an AAC system will keep them from acquiring speech.

It is important to understand that some children with ASD do not acquire speech; current estimates suggest this is true for 10%–30% of affected children. The great majority of children with ASD who are going to talk will do so by age 6. The chances that speech will emerge are much less after that age, although it's not impossible. Pickett, Pulara, O'Grady, and Barry (2009) found 167 reported cases of children with ASD who acquired speech between 5 and 13 years old, and there are surely other cases that have not been reported. It is not known why some children with ASD don't acquire speech. It may have to do with the precision of motor skills necessary to produce it. It may involve difficulty in making sense of or remembering the auditory signals that carry speech information so that the child is unable to establish a stable mental representation, or auditory image, of words in mind and cannot reproduce them through speech. It may be that some children with ASD never reach the "Aha!" moment that allows them to understand the purpose of speech. An AAC system that allows these children to express a range of messages is especially important. It will be the job of the SLP to

- Assess the child and family's need for an AAC system

- Choose an AAC system appropriate for the child and acceptable to the family

- Help the child and family learn to use the AAC system while continuing to emphasize, encourage, and practice speech.

Each component of the SLP's job with AAC includes the family because communication is always a two-way street. Children need a way to express themselves, but adults also need to understand and validate the child's form of communication. If the child is using signs as an AAC mode, then that means that people in the family and people in the neighborhood, as in Juan's case, need to know how and be willing to use the communication system along with the child. A child won't have as much success with a communication system that isn't embraced by others. Many AAC clinicians suggest that the family not only respond to AAC communication that the child produces, but also that they use the system themselves—signing when they talk to the child who signs, using pictures to accompany their speech for a child who uses pictures, or sending their messages on the iPad for a child who uses an iPad. The AAC's value will be enhanced when it is seen as an interactive exchange rather than a mechanical tool only the child uses.

Young children who adopt an AAC system should still receive some structured therapy to encourage speech. For example, the SLP may spend some time working with the child and family on using the AAC device and on teaching others in the child's world to use it, but also spend part of the time on activities that focus on speech. Speech is the most difficult form of communication to learn, and the brain is finely tuned to learn it only during the early years. It's that special talent for learning speech that is lost with age, which makes it so hard to acquire a foreign language and its unique accent once childhood has passed. If children with ASD are going to talk, then it is most likely that they will do so by the time they are 6 years old. If they don't learn by then, then their chances of acquiring speech are much reduced. Even though using an AAC system doesn't prevent a child from talking, children with ASD still need some special help in learning to do what other children do completely naturally and without effort, and talking is one of those things.

Some special techniques are needed to teach speech to children with ASD. Several methods have shown some success in getting preschoolers who are preverbal and have ASD to talk, and they will be briefly mentioned next. See Chapters 6 and 7 for more information about these methods.

ABA or discrete trial instruction (DTI) is the most common method for teaching speech to children with ASD. DTI uses a stimulus-response-reinforcement sequence to get a child to imitate sounds and words by rewarding productions that move closer to a correct target production. A long series of studies showed these methods can be quite effective for getting children who are preverbal and have ASD to talk. One addition to DTI for speech that seems to be helpful is the use of rapid motor imitation antecedent (RMIA) training, which gets the child to repeat a series of simple motor imitations before a vocal imitation (Tsiouri & Paul, 2012). DTI methods don't work for everyone, but one study showed they worked for about half the preschoolers with no speech in a clinical trial (Paul, Campbell, Tsiouri, & Gilbert, 2013).

Several other studies showed that some proportion of young children who are nonverbal and have ASD learn to talk using a method called *milieu teaching* (e.g., Paul et al., 2013; Yoder & Stone, 2006) or other naturalistic behavioral methods that are not as highly structured than DTI. These methods set up temptations like those used in assessment and require children to produce sounds and then speech in order to get objects and activities they enjoy. This method involves engineering the child's environment so that there is a lot of interesting stuff around, but the child can't gain access to it without help from the adult.

Finally, research by Kasari et al. (2014) showed that using an electronic device that generates speech—such as a switch, other devices that can be programmed to play prerecorded speech when activated, or software for tablet-style computers such as iPads that talks when a picture is touched—can also increase spoken language, especially when combined with milieu-style temptation activities.

Families of young children who are preverbal and have ASD should make use of AAC methods to provide the children with a way to express wants and needs and to begin to understand the function of communication during the early years. Some regular part of the communication program, however, should also include time devoted to modeling and eliciting speech, using one of the methods mentioned here. A child's opportunities to make the important transition from communication to language will be optimized when both an AAC modality and time to focus on vocal and speech production are provided.

A child's opportunities to make the important transition from communication to language will be optimized when both an AAC modality and time to focus on vocal and speech production are provided.

These interventions won't look like typical speech-language therapy, because they aren't focused on proper pronunciation or oral postures needed to produce sounds. Instead, their aim is to connect vocal sounds with functional communication. The link between sound and meaning is likely to be missing for children who are preverbal and have ASD; the problem is not simply that they do not know how to form the sounds of speech. They may not know how to form sounds, but the reason is probably not based in motor weakness or incoordination but in lack of practice that comes from not understanding the communicative function of making sounds. Once a child has the "Aha!" experience that communication is a way to get enjoyable things, it makes more sense to focus attention on the mechanics of speaking; that's the moment that needs to be created. Simple, consistent models of speech that the child can associate with fun activities need to be provided so that the desire to ask to do them again is created. It's why a child like Juan may start saying "ee" when he wants to eat after he's been taught the sign for eat. Once he sees the link between the sign, what he wants, and the word *eat,* he has a reason to learn to say "eat." Some children may take this additional step—to spontaneously say words they've learned through an AAC system. Additional opportunities to try spoken versions of communicative acts in supportive situations can enhance the chances that this transition to speech will take place, so some speech-focused activities need to be added to the sessions that involve working on an AAC system. Children need opportunities to practice the motor patterns involved in speech, because speech is a motor behavior that has to be learned through practice, just like other motor behaviors such as learning to ski, skate, or play an instrument. Words need to be connected to meaning, so the focus of intervention should not be solely on drilling motor patterns. Meaningful opportunities need to be provided so children with ASD can practice producing words and sounds in settings where immediate rewards are received.

WHAT CAN PARENTS DO TO SUPPORT
COMMUNICATION DEVELOPMENT IN YOUNG CHILDREN WITH ASD?

Although you certainly want to get your child with ASD into an intervention program as early as possible, there are many informal ways you can support your child's communicative development outside of formal therapy.

Communication

Most parents feel that they need the professionals to teach their child with ASD the important skills he or she needs to learn. It's true that there are some special techniques that are useful in working with children with ASD, and it does take extra patience to explicitly teach the things most children learn naturally without any effort or direct instruction. Many of the social communication skills a young child needs can be practiced in simple, everyday situations if you know how to take advantage of them. It is possible to identify situations in which you can slightly modify the way you behave or slightly alter the environment in order to contrive more situations for your child to practice communicating needs and ideas.

Parents often interpret their children's needs before they express them, but this can lead to missing opportunities to have children practice expressing thoughts in a conventional way. For example, when your child sees you pulling your telephone out of your bag and immediately runs toward you and looks at the telephone, you may know he or she wants the telephone to play Angry Birds. But instead of just handing over the telephone, you might say, "Oh, do you want something?" and pause and wait for the child to respond in some way. If you get a look and perhaps a sound or a sign, then you can turn over the tele-

phone, knowing your child has made a connection between expressing a communication and its result. If you can't elicit a request, and the child merely continues to look at the telephone or grabs at it, then you could take his or her hand, shape it into a point toward the telephone, make the sign for telephone, or offer a spoken prompt ("Telephone, please?"), depending on your child's current level of expression. You might give three chances to take your cue and produce a conventional request. If you don't get a request after

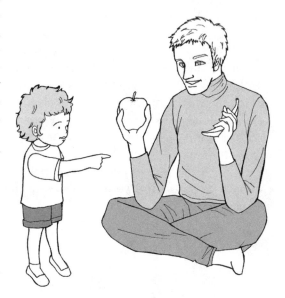

three attempts, then you can hand over the phone, first modeling "Telephone, please," or making the sign for the child.

These kinds of communication temptations can be embedded throughout your normal daily routines and include making requests as well as making choices (e.g., "Do you want the grapes or the blueberries?"), following a sequence (e.g., "First socks, then shoes"), playing hide-and-seek games (e.g., putting objects the child likes under covers and modeling how to exclaim "ball" when it's uncovered), and imitating actions (e.g., start a preferred routine game such as "The Itsy-Bitsy Spider" and pause, waiting for the child to imitate the last action before you produce the next one). You should feel free to ask your team for suggestions for including these kinds of communication temptations throughout your day. Once you start, you will discover many opportunities on your own to practice interactive abilities, and the more chances your child gets to use them, the more easily communication will come.

Eye Contact

You've probably heard and noticed that making eye contact is a primary difficulty for children with ASD. It's not that children with ASD never look people in the eye, but they do it less often and less skillfully. They are less likely to look not only at people but also at what other people look at, and they interpret other people's gaze patterns less adeptly. We don't want to simply get children to make eye contact, we want them to use gaze to organize their social interactions. You might try the following to help them:

- Hold items you are talking about to the child at eye level.

- Wait for the child to look at you before starting a communicative exchange or before giving an item he or she is requesting. For example, if your child is on a swing, then pull the swing close to you and don't let the swing go until the child looks at you.

- Play games such as hiding treasure in one of your closed fists, and have your child guess which hand it's in as you look back and forth from the child to the correct hand. Do the same with other locations, always looking back and forth from the child to the location to cue the correct place to look.

Reading

Looking at picture books is a great way to spend time with young children because it teaches them about how books work, which helps them get ready to read, and provides repetitive language that goes with attractive pictures, which helps them learn what words and sentences mean. It helps children at somewhat higher levels of development learn to remember and understand sequences of events in stories and talk about characters' feelings and intentions. They can also learn new words from books that they may not hear in everyday conversation. There's a lot to be gained from this simple and enjoyable activity.

Children with ASD often are less interested in books than other children. You may have to make the books a little more exciting for them than you would for another child by using funny voices, singing some of the words, or doing actions that go with the story. Numerous storybook apps are available on many electronic platforms that might appeal to your child. A good place to look for these is http://appadvice.com/applists/show/children-ipad-books.

Numerous storybook apps are available on many electronic platforms that might appeal to your child. A good place to look for these is http://appadvice.com/applists/show/children-ipad-books.

You might want to focus on using books to help children who already understand a lot of language comprehend how people feel, how they think, and how sometimes they don't mean exactly what they say. For example, put sticky notes with thought bubbles on the pages and ask your child what the character may be thinking.

Finding time to spend with books is a good investment, regardless of your child's level of function. Try to find ways of making storybook reading a special, fun time for your child, not a chore. You want to instill a love of books, and if you just can't find a way for your child to enjoy it, then it's better to let it go and try again another time. But children with ASD love routines, and if you can establish a predictable routine for reading a book together the same time every day in the same place, then your child will come to look forward to it. Try not to read the same book every time, or your child may become fixated on that book and not allow you to read others. There's no problem with returning often to a favorite book, however, as long as you can get the child to tolerate others as well.

How to Play with Your Child with ASD

Children love when their parents play with them, but remember that it only stays enjoyable for your child if you play at your child's level. Making a game more complicated than a child is ready for, even though it makes it more interesting for you, can frustrate the child. The following are some tips for playing with your child with ASD.

Repetitive Play Most children, especially those with ASD, love to play the same game repeatedly. This is one situation where you can use your child's enjoyment of repetition to advantage. Encourage reenacting the same sequence or game as often as the child likes (you will probably get tired of it before the child does), but add a little change in the routine every now and then. For example, if your child likes switching the light switch on and off, then make it into a game, but insist on taking turns. Let the child flick the switch, flick it once yourself, then put your hand over it and wait. When the child looks at you, say, "My turn," or "On," and try to get a vocal or motor request before letting him or her have a turn to flick. Again, give up to three chances to follow the prompt. If the child responds, then let him or her flick the switch a few times; if not, then give one more prompt and let him or her have a turn. Repeat until the child tires of the game.

Play with Toys   Children with ASD often like cause-and-effect toys, such as Poppin' Pals or a jack-in-the-box. These are fine for repetitive play, but you may want to encourage your child to use other toys as well, which will likely require you, or perhaps the child's siblings, to play along. Educational toys, such as shape sorters, nesting and stacking toys, and puzzles, are worth including because they help the child learn spatial concepts and can also serve as a way to introduce the words for shapes, colors, and sizes. If the child isn't initially interested in them, then try playing with them yourself (or having the sibling play) for a bit and let the child do as he or she likes. It's likely he or she will become interested in what you have. If so, you can use the toy to take turns, and you can name the colors, shapes, and sizes of the objects as you play with them (e.g., "I'm putting the square in now. The blue square. Your turn. Here's the circle. You put the circle in.") Keep all the pieces yourself so the child needs to interact with you to get each piece and take a turn. If the child doesn't spontaneously join the play, then you can move other objects out of reach and suggest the child join you or the sibling. Remember that this only works if the result is fun for the child. If he or she protests and becomes upset about losing access to what he or she was doing, don't worry. Let it go and try again another time.

Don't forget the play value of things that children with typical development often treat as toys, even when they weren't meant that way. The cardboard box a toy was packaged in can often provide as much enjoyment as the toy itself. Your child may like to climb into a large cardboard "bus" and be pushed. The cardboard box can become a bumpy bus, a fast train, or a rocky boat, all of which can be used to teach your child to request which vehicle he or she wants after a few turns.

It is especially important for children with ASD to learn to enjoy a variety of objects and activities so they don't become fixated on any one. Even if you find something your child loves, be sure to vary it in some way over time. Continue to introduce new play things and model different ways to use them. Siblings are great at this because activities with another child are often appealing even to children with ASD.

Letter and Number Play   Many children with ASD seem particularly interested in letters and numbers. They may want to repeatedly put together the same alphabet puzzle or line up numbered blocks in the same sequence many times. Parents can become excited about this kind of play and encourage it, thinking it bodes well for reading and math abilities. It may, but it can also develop into an isolated or *splinter* skill that fails to lead to adaptive use.

If you notice this kind of interest in your child, then try to encourage variety. If the child likes an alphabet puzzle, then try encouraging matching each letter piece to a plastic magnet letter (the kind that stick on the refrigerator), letters in an alphabet book, or letters on T-shirts. Use the letters to sing the alphabet song together, putting the pieces on the table instead of in the puzzle. Stack the letters as if they were blocks, get a bucket and take turns playing basketball by throwing each letter in the bucket. Play Hide and Seek by taking turns putting each letter in different places around the room and letting the child find it. This would also be an opportunity to either look at where you hid the letter to help the child find it (and to help him or her learn to follow others' gaze), to point to where you hid it (to help him or her learn to follow a point), or—if your child understands some language—to say where it is (e.g., "Look under the table"). Feel free to name the letter in each activity or say, "A is for apple," but the point is to help the child learn new ways to play instead of constantly repeating the same ways. It's certainly possible to learn the letter names and sounds this way, but this kind of play will also lead to learning a more flexible set of play schemes that can be used with other materials. Try introducing some other materials into these games whenever your child will accept them. Box 3.4 presents some additional tips for playing with your child with ASD.

 Playing with Your Child with ASD

- Try to have 5–10 minutes each day set aside for play. Your child doesn't have to have the same playmate each time (e.g., mom, dad, brother, sister, cousin, grandma).

- Sit at your child's level (e.g., on the floor).

- Let your child choose the toys or activities and follow his or her lead.

- Imitate what your child does by doing the same thing next to him or her and take turns (e.g., he or she pushes the car once, then take it from him or her, do the same action, and hand it back).

- Slow down your rate of speech and vary your volume and pitch in a sing-song way. Or just pick a tune and sing whatever you say.

- Talk about what your child is doing in short and simple words or sentences.

- Do not expect your child to repeat what you say.

- Tell your child the names of objects instead of asking him or her to label them.

- Try to avoid saying "no."

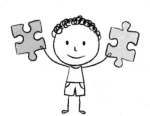

(continued)

BOX 3.4 *(continued)*

- Use the child's name at the end of a sentence, especially when praising him or her (e.g., "Well done, Ahmed!").

- Allow silent times.

- Wait for your child to begin interactions.

- Understand and respond to any form of communication, even a simple quick look at you while he or she is playing. Respond with, "Yes, I see you playing with the car!"

- Treat behavior as if it were communication, even if the child may not have meant it that way. If the child accidentally rolls a car in your direction, then take it and say, "Oh my turn! Thank you! You gave me a turn!"

- Imitate and praise any sounds the child makes, especially those that sound like speech. Don't worry if you don't understand what the child meant or if he or she meant anything. Respond to his or her sounds with excitement and your own vocalization.

- If the child says a word, then repeat it back with correct pronunciation, but continue to respond to his or her immature form with your mature form.

- Praise your child lavishly, using facial expressions, hugs, tickles, or anything else he or she likes.

- Ignore any inconsequential behaviors while playing (e.g., if he or she screams when blocks fall apart). If you give attention to these behaviors, even by trying to calm him or her down, then they may actually be strengthened. Simply help him or her fix it without any comment or facial expression.

- Keep it happy. If your child becomes upset at something you try, then ignore the outburst and go back to the previous form of play. Don't give up; try again later.

- Set the scene for some messy play. Cover the table with plastic and let the child fingerpaint with pudding, shaving cream, or cornstarch paste. This is a great chance to use words for how things feel—*slippery, gooey, yucky, cold, sticky,* and so forth.

CONCLUSION

This chapter discussed the central place that communication has in identifying and treating ASD in young children and explained how this crucial skill is evaluated as part of the assessment of children with ASD. It also looked at some of the approaches to treating the communication impairments common in young children with the syndrome. Finally, the chapter provided ideas about how you can supplement the formal intervention program your child will receive with simple activities that can be included within everyday routines. The next chapter introduces you to the professionals who may be involved in developing and delivering the more formal part of your child's intervention program.

What Types of Professionals Work with Children with Autism Spectrum Disorder?

Neddy is 4 years old, and he was diagnosed with ASD just before his third birthday. He has been receiving early intervention services for the last 18 months. Neddy also has epilepsy and is under the supervision of a neurologist. He is verbal and uses two- to three-word sentences to communicate his needs. In addition to his difficulties with communication, Neddy has some difficulties with transitions; dressing, feeding, and toileting have all been a struggle. The early intervention team who assessed him recommended that he receive speech-language therapy, occupational therapy, home-based early intervention, and physical therapy. A neurologist who specializes in childhood seizure disorders also monitors him. Neddy has been making progress during the last 6 months, and his parents are pleased that he is beginning to interact more and use language to talk about what he sees. His understanding of language also has improved, although he still repeats whole phrases from his favorite books and movies.

Neddy's feeding is one of the issues of concern for his family. He had always been a picky eater and only ate a handful of foods, but more recently he is refusing what he normally would eat. When Neddy's OT, Laura, came to visit, Neddy's mom told her how concerned she was, "He is refusing to eat anything new. He normally eats creamed potatoes with cheese and carrots, but when I tried using a different cheese, he refused to eat it. Now when I give him the same creamed potatoes with the same cheese he ate before, he either turns his head away or spits it out. I don't know what to do. He already has such a limited diet, and he can't survive on grapes, scrambled eggs, and one type of cake." Laura suggested that she would speak to Kate, Neddy's SLP, and they would together think about how they could address Neddy's feeding difficulties.

Laura and Kate met and discussed that the first step should be conducting a functional behavioral assessment (FBA) to establish why Neddy was struggling so much with feeding, and they would discuss this at their next team meeting. After a week of collecting data it was apparent that Neddy's feeding behavior was primarily due to his difficulties communicating how he feels about the different foods. The team suggested to Neddy's family that they break the feeding down into steps and introduce new foods to Neddy through play. They also decided to use a visual tool to help Neddy communicate how he feels about the different foods, and Neddy's early intervention special educator would have snack time with him in order to get the program started. The physical therapist (PT) would be consulted about positioning during feeding to be sure Neddy was comfortable while eating.

You will likely be introduced to a bewildering array of professionals when your child is diagnosed with ASD, each of whom has a role to play in helping your child develop. As your child makes the transition from the diagnostic assessment process to intervention, services may be provided by a team of professionals, perhaps different from the assessment group. This chapter discusses the different professionals you may meet, their roles, and how their services fit into your child's overall program.

In the preceding example, the team worked together with Neddy's family to identify the underlying reasons for Neddy's feeding problems. Professionals shared their expertise, but they understood how important it was to work as a team because of the overlap in their skills and shared goals. Although this is time consuming and hard to coordinate, the benefits are well worth the effort. You can take an active role in making sure this kind of collaboration happens for your child. Ideas for facilitating the collaboration are discussed at the end of this chapter. The roles of the different professionals who may be involved in your child's treatment and their qualifications, areas of expertise, and overlap in skills are discussed next. As you get to know the various professionals who will participate in your child's intervention, you may want to ask about their knowledge and experience in working with children with ASD. This chapter introduces you to the following professionals:

- Speech-language pathologists (SLP)
- Occupational therapists (OT)
- Physical therapists (PT)
- Board certified behavior analysts (BCBAs)
- Special educators/early interventionists (SPED/EI)
- Social workers
- Educational aides/paraprofessionals
- Physicians

SPEECH-LANGUAGE PATHOLOGISTS

As we've seen, difficulty in social-communication—the ability to understand and send messages to others—is a core impairment in ASD. SLPs are trained to assess and treat disorders of speech, language, and communication. Although SLP is the term preferred by these professionals, people also sometimes refer to them as speech therapists, speech pathologists, or speech teachers. All these terms are used to refer to the same set of practitioners. SLPs in the United States are required to hold a master's degree from an educational program accredited by the Council on Academic Accreditation in Audiology and Speech-Language Pathology in order to obtain their certification to practice from the American Speech-Language-Hearing Association (ASHA; www.asha.org). SLPs are trained to assess, diagnose, and treat disorders related to speech, language, communication, voice (e.g., hoarseness), swallowing, feeding, and fluency (e.g., stuttering). Some SLPs have specialized training in autism or behavior analysis. The terms SLPs use to discuss ASD's core impairments are reviewed next. Then we'll talk about the role of the SLP in your child's program.

Communication

As we discussed in Chapter 2, *communication* is the umbrella term used to refer to sending a message, in any form, between a sender and a receiver. It includes not only talking but also reading, writing, and using signs, pictures, body language, and facial expressions; even the way one dresses communicates a message to people from the same culture. Animals communicate too, with each other and with people (e.g., when your dog whines and looks at you and the door to be let outside) (see Chapter 2). Infants communicate, as well, before they learn to talk. They smile to get people to pay attention to them, make sounds in back-and-forth babbling that has the same structure as conversation, and show off when they learn that particular actions get others to look or laugh. These early forms of communication help the infant learn how to use communicating to secure enjoyable experiences and they lay the foundation for language development.

Communication intervention aims to help children learn to express their wants, needs, thoughts, and feelings in ways that are understandable and acceptable within their community. Sometimes children with ASD develop maladaptive means of communicating; they may bang their head when they are frustrated or push another child when they want his or her toy. Communication intervention provides more adaptive ways to express these intentions. It may be through speech, such as teaching the child to say, "Stop it," rather than biting if another child is annoying. Communication intervention can also involve nonspeech forms (e.g., AAC) for children who have trouble using verbal communication, as we saw in Chapter 3. We'll talk more about this issue in the Speech section.

Language

We talked in Chapter 2 about the fact that although animals communicate, they don't use language. Language is a special form of communication that follows rules and allows humans to get across an infinite variety of messages. The rules of language tell us how to put meaningful units (words) together to enable the creation of sentences that have never been said before and also make it possible to string together several ideas to convey complex thoughts ("Four score and seven years ago our fathers brought forth on this continent, a new nation, conceived in Liberty, and dedicated to the proposition that all men are created equal"). In addition, the rules allow for a variation in the meaning of sentences depending on the word order ("The dog bit the man" versus "The man bit the dog"). Children typically learn most of these rules and many of the words they can use between 1 and 5 years of age. The process of learning language is usually delayed in children with ASD, as we've seen. Language intervention is almost always appropriate for these children. It involves first teaching the child to understand and use words, signs, or other symbols. These are usually taught individually at first by associating the word or sign with the picture or object to which it refers. The child is later taught to combine the words and signs into phrases (e.g., "my shoe," "big cookie") and then sentences that follow the grammatical rules of the language of the school and family. Once children with ASD learn the basic rules of grammar, they almost always need additional help in the pragmatic aspects of language, the rules for using language appropriately in social settings. For example, they may need practice using different ways of talking depending on whom they are addressing—a friend ("Hi, how are ya?") or a new adult acquaintance ("How do you do? My name is Malik Jones").

Speech

Human beings have highly evolved specialized structures for expressing language in the form of speech. As we explained in Chapter 2, speech is the production of language by means of articulating sounds with the vocal cords, tongue, teeth, and lips. Speech therapy refers to helping children learn to say the sounds of speech correctly for their language environment. Many children, including children with ASD, have trouble correctly pronouncing sounds during the preschool years, often producing amusing errors such as those made by a little girl who called her brother's troop the "tub stouts" instead of "cub scouts" when she was a toddler. Speech therapy is usually reserved for those preschoolers who don't just make errors but whose speech is so hard for others to understand that they become frustrated. Older children who continue to have trouble making certain sounds in the school years also may receive speech therapy.

Some forms of speech therapy are provided to children with ASD who don't produce any speech at all in order to elicit first speech production. There is disagreement among SLPs, however, as to whether to focus on teaching children how to make speech sounds using speech units, or *phonemes,* or working directly on words. Those who use words as the target accept productions that approximate the intended word.

AAC therapy is another approach that may be used with children who do not produce any speech. Forms of AAC include signs and systems using pictures on cards or on a screen (e.g., Blisssymbols, Mayer-Johnson Picture Symbols, and the Picture Exchange Communication System [PECS] are some examples; see Chapter 7). Some children who don't speak may be able to learn to use symbols or writing to express themselves. Although these symbol and writing systems were originally developed for children with typical cognitive development who have severe motor disorders that impair speech production (e.g., cerebral palsy), some children with ASD have been able to master them. Technological AAC systems are now easily accessible through apps on consumer electronic devices that translate typing or chosen picture symbols into spoken language. These text-to-speech apps are inexpensive and easy to access on smartphones and tablets, but they do require the child to master the motor and cognitive skills involved in typing, spelling, and language formulation. Unfortunately, not every child who does not speak is able to make use of them.

Role of the Speech-Language Pathologist

An SLP may be the first professional to evaluate a child with ASD because many parents of toddlers with ASD are concerned when their child fails to start talking when other toddlers do. Communication in all its forms is so central to autism that SLPs will almost always be part of the diagnostic and treatment teams.

The SLP will assess the various skills that contribute to communication during the diagnostic process and periodically throughout the treatment, often simultaneously working on several skills. The SLP may provide services in the home, classroom, child care center, or community setting. The SLP will want to observe you and your child together as part of the diagnostic evaluation to determine how he or she responds to communicative bids with familiar people and to collect information through review of your child's medical and educational records, questionnaires and interviews with family and teachers, and the administration of standardized tests and less formal assessment probes. In treatment, the SLP may work directly with your child or in a coaching capacity to help you and the child's other teachers and caregivers implement strategies that enhance communication. The SLP also will plan treatment goals and review progress with other team members.

The areas addressed in treatment and the materials used by the SLP during the early years may overlap with those used by other team members, because communication is a basic building block for all learning and will need to be incorporated into many of the child's activities. For example, the OT and the SLP may both use water play, playdough, bubbles, or a container filled with beans. The SLP, however, may use the bubbles to encourage and teach your child to request with simple words such as *open* or *bubbles*. The OT may use the same activity to teach your child how to hold the wand appropriately or how to manage discomfort and desensitize overreactions around a feeling of wetness caused by popping bubbles. You will have a chance to talk about your priorities for therapy during meetings when your child's program is discussed with the team, and you and the team will decide together how your priorities can be integrated into the program. The following vignette describes a home-based SLP session and some of the skills taught by the SLP.

Bonnie is an SLP providing home care services to Emma, who is almost 3 years old. Emma uses fewer than 10 words expressively and her understanding is at the level of a 2 year old. She is exploratory in her play and enjoys some simple cause-and-effect activities such as popping bubbles, emptying containers, and throwing a ball. She is, however, repetitive in play, with a limited range of interests and often requests to watch the same Beyoncé video repeatedly. She has difficulty attending to other activities for more than a few minutes. Bonnie has introduced playing with playdough to help Emma develop expressive and receptive language as well as attention and play skills. Emma likes the texture, and rolling and squeezing the playdough also enables her to work on her fine motor skills. Bonnie has been able to encourage Emma to sit at the table, and she has noticed that Emma's attention also has improved. She also noticed that after she names colors of playdough for Emma as she plays that Emma has started spontaneously naming some of the colors. Now when Bonnie says, "Take the green playdough," Emma will quickly select the correct color. She also has been able to introduce Emma to finger-puppets. Emma enjoys hearing Bonnie talk for the puppets in funny voices and responds when a puppet asks her to follow a simple direction. Emma has even started giving simple directions to the puppets, such as "jump." Emma's mother has noticed that when they play on the trampoline together, Emma also uses her approximation of *jump* to ask for another turn on the trampoline.

Bonnie was not only able to teach Emma to understand new words and produce new sounds, but there were also several developmental domains she was able to work on at the same time. Bonnie was able to work on Emma's gross and fine motor imitation skills, attention skills, and play skills by using an activity involving playdough.

The SLP may collaborate with teachers and other professionals to provide strategies and additional materials to supplement objectives within the treatment plan. For example, your child may be exhibiting some interfering behaviors and the BCBA and SLP may see that your child would benefit from a checklist, or pictures to communicate needs. SLPs collaborate with OTs to work on feeding skills and preferences for children who have difficulty with food intake. Table 4.1 provides a list of terms and definitions that SLPs use in working with children with ASD.

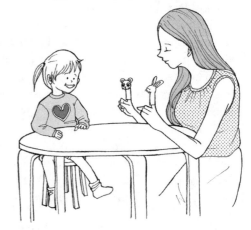

OCCUPATIONAL THERAPISTS

An OT is a health care professional with a degree from an educational program accredited by the American Occupational Therapy Association (AOTA; http://www.aota.org) who works with people of all ages to improve performance of activities of daily living (ADLs) and adaptive behaviors. For young children with developmental disorders and learning disabilities, this typically means working on play skills, self-care, and fine motor skills such as writing or drawing. Although children with ASD have primary difficulties with their speech, language, and communication skills, many have additional challenges with their sensory perception, motor skills, and daily living activities. The OT working with your child will use functional activities to help him or her develop skills needed to participate in everyday life, learning, and leisure activities. Functional activities can include bathing, feeding, dressing, and other naturally occurring routines that serve a purpose.

Current best practice is to have the OT work alongside teachers, with other professionals, or in the home with parents in order to model the therapeutic activities that can be integrated into daily routines. OTs and other service providers who work within an educational setting collaborate with the teachers, providing services within the classroom (sometimes referred to as pushing-in or collaborative teaching) rather than pulling a child out for individual therapy in a less inclusive setting. The purpose is to enhance instruction in the classroom content and core curricular goals while practicing the targeted skills during authentic peer interactions. If the OT works within a home setting, then he or she may work alongside the SLP, early intervention teacher, or BCBA. Some OT goals may include

- Promoting independence in skills that require fine motor and hand-to-eye coordination for ADLs (also often referred to as self-help or adaptive skills), such as dressing, bathing, toileting, using utensils for feeding, grasping toys, and using a crayon, pen, or pencil.

- Helping children manage sensitivities. Children can either be hyper- (above average) or hypo- (below average) sensitive to information received through any of the five senses. Children may be highly reactive to touch/textures, levels of sound, certain smells or tastes, or light. Or their sensitivity may be very low and put them at risk of danger for harm (e.g., listening to extremely loud music, eye damage from staring at bright lights, other injury due to a high pain threshold). The most evidence-based practice for this purpose is systematic de-sensitization, which we illustrated with the vacuum cleaner example in Chapter 2. Other strategies OTs may employ include:

  - Teaching cognitive and comprehension skills through movement and related gross motor activities.

  - Assessing and reducing environmental barriers that limit a child's participation in family, learning, and community-based activities. This could

Table 4.1. Skill areas speech-language pathologists (SLPs) assess and treat

Skill area	Explanation	Example
Receptive language skills	These skills relate to the understanding of spoken communication, gestures, and written language.	Jacob is learning the names of everyday objects. In the morning when getting dressed, Jacob's mother asks him to select different items of clothing placed on his bed.
Expressive language	This is the ability to communicate using words, gestures, or symbols. This includes how words or gestures are combined, range of vocabulary, and number of words the child knows. It also includes syntax (sentence structures) children use and their use of morphology (grammatical structures).	Jacob is learning to request a variety of items throughout the day using approximation of spoken words paired with the gesture. Jacob's mother encourages him to request during mealtimes and bath time when he is highly motivated. She is working on teaching Jacob to request for *bubbles, up, open, eat,* and *juice.*
Pragmatics	This area involves the use of language and nonverbal communication. This also includes some of the hidden social rules, sometimes referred to as the hidden curriculum, that are not always naturally understood by individuals with autism spectrum disorder and vary according to gender and culture. This could be using eye contact, knowing how to greet familiar and unfamiliar adults, knowing the appropriate distance when standing with a communicative partner, or knowing where to stand in an elevator and what to say and what not to say.	When requesting bubbles, Jacob's mother holds the bubbles by her eyes to encourage Jacob to look at her before she blows the bubbles to him.
Play behaviors	These are how and what the child uses as objects to pretend, which is related to the ability to use words to stand for things and how to use language and communication skills during play with adults and other children.	Jacob is learning to imitate what others do with objects. Jacob's mother is teaching him how to imitate different actions with objects during bath time (e.g., pushing a small boat in the water).
Articulation of sounds	This is producing the sounds for language. The SLP will assess which sounds the child uses and how the child combines these sounds to produce words that can be understood by others.	Jacob makes a lot of sounds when he is on the swing at the playground. His mother has started to repeat some of these sounds back to Jacob. The team has noticed that Jacob is making more sounds when he plays.
Oral-motor functioning	This is how the child is able to control and coordinate the gross and fine motor movements of the mouth, including the tongue, lips, and jaw.	Jacob is being encouraged to hold a cup and drink a variety of liquids.
Voice	This area covers voice quality and its control in relation to the use of pitch, loudness, and fluency. Some children with autism spectrum disorder come across as having a monotone voice or a squeaky, high-pitched voice, which may be caused by an inability to control their voice quality.	When Jacob is singing children's songs he is encouraged to copy the actions and fill in some of the key phrases of the songs and adjust his loudness (e.g., singing "Row, Row, Row Your Boat" quietly and loudly).
Verbal memory	This is the child's ability to recall information received through language. Some children with autism have well-developed verbal memory systems and are able to recall phrases from movies and video games; however, they do not necessarily understand what they recall.	Jacob likes to play on the iPad and he listens to "Head, Shoulders, Knees, and Toes." He was able to change the settings on the iPad when he was 3 years old so that he could listen to the song in multiple languages. He was able to sing the song in English, Japanese, and Spanish.
Attention	This is the length of time the child is able to sustain focus on meaningful stimuli, especially language. Some children find it easier to sustain their attention for activities that are exploratory or sensory (e.g., playing with water, filling and dumping sand). They may be able to do this for up to an hour if left on their own; however, they may have difficulty sitting on the carpet in preschool for storytime.	Jacob is able to sustain his attention for longer during bath time because it is an exploratory activity. Jacob finds it difficult to concentrate for more than a few minutes when he is being read a simple bedtime story.

involve special seating or carrel-like barriers to block out visual distraction during one-to-one teaching times.

- Supporting and preparing children to make transitions between activities, from one place to another, or from home-based services to preschool, preschool to school, and/or other community-based programs.

An OT will generally assess your child in the following areas:

Strength, Range of Motion, and Muscle Tone   The child's overall body strength and muscle tone is assessed as well as his or her range of motion. Range of motion is the amount of mobility available at each joint. Some children with ASD have low muscle tone, which affects their ability to sit, hold utensils, and conduct simple ADLs such as removing socks.

Fine Motor and Gross Motor Skills and Balance   Fine motor skills use the small muscles of the hands and feet. Fine motor skills generally refer to hand skills because hands are used for more skilled tasks. Some children with ASD have difficulty with fine motor skills such as buttoning, zipping up clothes, or opening containers. Gross motor skills use the larger muscles of the body such as those necessary to run, jump, hop, skip, and throw or catch a ball. These affect balance, too, which refers to maintaining upright posture during standing, sitting, and walking. A child with poor balance may have difficulty standing on one leg to be able to put on a pair of pants.

Bilateral Motor Coordination   Coordinating the two sides of the body may be underdeveloped in some children with ASD, which can affect ADLs and scholastic skills. A child first coordinates the use of the two sides of his or her body symmetrically. This is typically seen in the ability to play hand games such as Pat-a-cake. The motor skills that accompany these social games may also be slow to develop because many children with ASD do not play these games when they are young due to difficulties developing social skills. Later in typical development, asymmetrical motor coordination develops to allow the two sides of the body to operate differently. These skills are needed for play activities such as climbing the ladder on a slide. Bilateral coordination skills lead to an awareness of the two sides of the body, which is necessary for right/left discrimination as well as selecting a preferred or dominant side, called *laterality,* which leads to handedness. Children with ASD who have motor incoordination or immaturity have an added layer of difficulties that, when combined with difficulty understanding language concepts, can lead to problems in school activities during gym class or playground games.

Sensory Processing   The ability to take in information through the senses and make meaningful responses based on sensory input often is impaired in children with ASD. OTs recognize seven senses, five that are external and two that are internal (see Table 4.2).

A child needs to use information derived from all senses effectively, both those senses that pick up input from the environment (vision, hearing, touch, smell, and taste) as well as those from one's own body (balance and proprioception). Children with ASD often have difficulty registering and making sense of sensory input. They may be overly sensitive to some sounds (e.g., crying at the sound of an electric toothbrush) and at the same time undersensitive to the sound of voices (e.g., fail to respond when their name is called). This difficulty managing sensory information can affect social adjustment. For example, a child with ASD may flap his or her hands in response to noisy stimuli, but this behavior may lead to stigmatizing by peers and negative responses from adults. The team working with your child, and the OT in particular, will provide suggestions to replace these maladaptive responses with more acceptable ways to manage sensitivity and regulate behavior. OTs may also provide desensitization activities to help the child gradually learn to tolerate displeasing stimuli.

Visual-Perceptual/Motor Skills   Visual-perceptual skills enable children to discriminate among drawn, written, and pictured forms and to judge their meaning. A number of specific skills generally fall into this category, including

- *Visual discrimination:* the ability to distinguish one visual pattern from another

- *Visual closure:* the ability to perceive a whole pattern when shown only parts of that pattern

- *Visual-motor coordination:* the ability to match motor output with visual input

Table 4.2.   The seven senses recognized by occupational therapists

Sense	Explanation
Visual	The ability to process information through the eyes and to make sense of spatial orientation and direction, color, shape, and intensity of light
Auditory	The perception of different sound wave frequencies through the ear, including loudness, pitch, localization of sounds, and discrimination
Tactile	This system is responsible for the sense of touch over the body's surface area and oral cavity, including the ability to discriminate between different textures and temperatures
Gustatory	The ability to taste and differentiate among sour, salty, bitter, and sweet tastes
Olfactory	The ability to detect odors and measure their intensity
Vestibular	Information to help detect and process one's sense of movement, the pull of earth's gravity, and the position of one's body in space
Proprioceptive	Feedback from senses about the effects of one's own motor actions (e.g., hearing oneself talk, seeing where one's hand is when the arm is raised)

Poor visual-motor integration can lead to problems with fine motor tasks that rely heavily on visual feedback, including threading laces, drawing, painting, building with blocks, playing computer games, and using a computer mouse.

Activities of Daily Living The focus of ADLs for young children with ASD is on self-care, play, and school tasks. Some children with ASD may have difficulty learning to use eating utensils, hold a cup, get dressed and undressed, take a shower/bath, use the toilet, and manipulate grooming and hygiene tools. Play activities, such as catching or throwing a ball may be problematic due to motor difficulties as well as difficulties understanding the rules of games. OTs and SLPs often run groups together in which the OT may focus on the motor skills and the SLP will focus on having the child make eye contact, take turns, and respond appropriately within the game. The need to learn tasks such as writing, keyboarding, using and organizing school tools, and being involved in group play may require additional assistance from OTs as children with ASD get older and move through the school years. Some areas of concern that often are the focus of OT intervention are

- Dressing: clothes on backward, shoes on wrong feet, difficulty buttoning, and tying laces

- Difficulty sequencing steps and initiating self-care

- Disliking necessary activities such as brushing teeth, putting body parts in water, and washing hair

- Pushing food off to the edge of the plate

- Messy and picky eating

- Avoidance of physical closeness and interactions with peers

- Frequent switching of the hand used either during a task or with different tasks

Some elements of OT practice are controversial, like many aspects of therapy for children with ASD. Although OTs typically work on developing adaptive skills and reducing sensory sensitivities through standard behavioral methods, there are some OT practices that are less well established in the scientific literature, including practices sometimes called sensory integration or sensory diets that may use special rooms with ball pits, twinkling lights, swings, or other equipment. Many children with ASD (as well as many typically developing children) enjoy the opportunity to swing or play in a ball pit. Other approaches may include brushing or massaging the child with ASD or having him or her wear a weighted vest. Some children with ASD enjoy these activities, and there may be no harm in using them if the child likes them. But it is important to understand that there is no evidence that these practices provide any benefits that extend beyond the immediate pleasure of engaging in them.

In other words, they don't teach the child skills. Although these practices are sometimes used to calm children who become upset, this too has its dangers. Such practices may inadvertently teach children that staging a meltdown is all that is needed to get out of a situation they dislike and get into a situation that they prefer. Families are encouraged to seek out OT services that focus on building skills for play, self-help, and academics and use behavioral methods to desensitize children who overreact to stimuli, rather than those that make use of these unproven practices.

PHYSICAL THERAPISTS

A PT is a health care professional who has received a graduate degree from a physical therapy program accredited by the American Physical Therapy Association (APTA; http://www.apta.org) before taking the national licensure exam allowing him or her to practice. A PT will assess your child for difficulties involving gross motor skills such as mobility, posture, and balance. Although most children with ASD have few difficulties with these gross motor skills, some do have experience challenges in these areas. PTs may work with very young children with ASD on basic motor skills such as sitting, rolling, standing, running, and climbing. These are important skills that are needed to develop other skills such as dressing and play. The PT may also work with the OT and SLP with children with ASD who have feeding difficulties. The PT will be able to assess and recommend the best position for the child to be in to maximize engagement in everyday activities. The PT may also recommend tools that can be used to support the child's mobility, such as special chairs and bolsters.

Some children with autism can have low muscle tone, even if they appear very active, and as a result show poor core muscle strength. They may also have balance issues, which can affect their ability to sit up, ride a bicycle, and pump their legs to swing. Most PTs who work with children with ASD work with them either in clinical settings and/or home settings. They may also work with parents to teach them techniques for helping their child build muscle strength, coordination, and skills.

A PT will often be one of the members of the early intervention team and may do a joint visit or therapy session with another therapist at home or in the community, as happened in Sam's case.

Samantha (known as Sam) is 28 months old and has been receiving early intervention services for the last 2 months from a team of specialists. When Alexander, the PT, and Veronica, the SLP, were visiting her at home, Sam's mother, Katie, expressed concern regarding Sam's difficulty sitting during bath times and mealtimes. "I'm finding lunchtime really hard. She used to sit on the sofa to eat, but we are now trying to get her to sit down for meals in a highchair. She can sit for a few minutes, but then she slumps and leans over to the right. At first I thought it was game or behavior but I realized it's not.

She is a good eater but it's almost as though she can't keep himself up. The same happens when it's bath time. She loves the water, and it is one of the best times to teach her to ask for things. She just finds it so hard to sit upright for any length of time, which makes playing in the water and with the bath toys really challenging. She loves listening to music in the park and throwing coins into the musicians' buckets, but it's so hard for her to stand and keep her balance."

Alexander explained that Sam's difficulties indicated low muscle and weak core muscle strength. Providing Sam with a special chair would help in the short term. Alexander also showed Katie and Veronica some games to play with Sam that were actually exercises to strengthen core muscles. They also agreed that Veronica would do a community visit to the park with Sam and her mom where she could show Katie how to support Sam in standing while Veronica worked with Katie on getting her to request coins to put in the musicians' bucket.

Alexander told Katie, "We want Sam to be comfortable and competent in her body so she can learn the other skills we are working on such as communication and play. Sam uses so much energy at the moment trying to sit up in the bath or stand upright in the park that she doesn't have the energy left to play. She can play with the toys now that she has a special chair, and you can work on teaching her to request the toys she wants. If one adult supports Sam's hips when she is in the park listening to music, then the other adult can help her ask for the coins that she loves to throw into the bucket."

PTs are more likely to come to a child's preschool or school as the child grows older. They may work on more complex playground skills, such as hopping, skipping, and ball skills (kicking, throwing, and catching a ball). Children's ability to play at the playground as they get older affects their opportunities to socialize with others, and this can be a difficult area for children with ASD. The PT may work with children to help them develop the necessary motor skills for the playground so they are more easily able to join in with peers' games. In addition, motor skills such as standing on one leg and being able to balance can affect independence for adaptive skills such as bathing, dressing, and feeding.

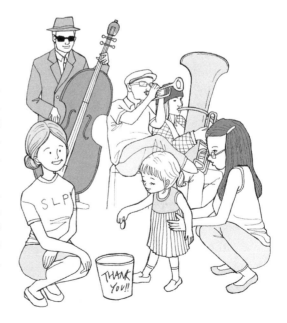

PTs who work in school settings will either pull children out to work with them one to one or collaborate in group settings such as gym/physical education and swim class.

BOARD CERTIFIED BEHAVIOR ANALYSTS

If you have a child with ASD, you might have heard a lot about Applied Behavior Analysis (ABA) and Functional Behavior Assessment (FBA). ABA is discussed in more detail in Chapters 6 and 7. This chapter talks about who delivers ABA instruction and what FBA contributes to your child's program.

ABA is a method of instruction that involves changing behavior through changing the antecedents (or what comes before a behavior happens) and consequences (what comes after a behavior happens). ABA is practiced by behavior analysts who are certified by a national organization, the Behavior Analyst Certification Board (http://www.bacb.com). A behavior analyst who meets the standards of this board is referred to as a Board Certified Behavior Analyst (BCBA). These standards include a master's degree with 225 graduate hours in behavior analysis and 750–1,500 hours of work experience supervised by a BCBA. Board Certified assistant Behavior Analysts (BCaBAs) hold a bachelor's degree with 135 hours of classroom instruction in behavior analysis and 500–1,000 hours of supervised work experience.

Apart from planning and implementing behavior therapy, a primary function of BCBAs is to conduct Functional Behavior Analysis (FBA). FBA involves gathering and analyzing information about a child's behavior and the circumstances that surround it in order to determine the purpose or intent of the child's actions. The assumption of FBA is that there is a reason maladaptive behaviors exist; they are governed (weakened or strengthened) by the consequences that follow them. BCBAs see behavior as a form of communication, so their goal is to figure out what message a particular behavior is sending. The maladaptive behavior may be the child's way of nonverbally saying, "I'm tired," "I'm bored," or "I'm upset." In other words, behavior serves a function. The goal of the FBA is to discover the function of a significant inappropriate or challenging behavior, such as aggression or self-injury. The FBA will help identify the circumstances that trigger (antecedent) or maintain (consequence) the challenging behavior and then assist in creating new triggers and consequences that will decrease it and increase new adaptive, productive, or proactive behaviors. Here's how it works. Behaviors usually function to accomplish one of two things:

1. To get something we want, such as

    •   Social positive reinforcement or attention

    •   Tangible reinforcement: access to goodies or reinforcing materials (food or toys)

    •   Automatic reinforcement: some intrinsic reward for the individual that the individual enjoys engaging in when left alone, such as humming

2. To avoid or escape something we don't like, such as pain, fear, boredom, or tasks that are difficult.

If benefits don't result from a behavior, then people usually stop doing it. So BCBAs try to learn what benefit (either a reward or an escape) a child is getting from a behavior, then manipulate either the antecedent (triggers) or the consequence (result) in order to reduce problem behaviors or increase desirable ones.

FBA typically consists of detailed observation of a child in the environment in which maladaptive behaviors happen. The BCBA will observe what happens just before and just after the maladaptive behavior in order to determine what triggers it and what benefits come from it. These observations, which may take several hours to complete, provide the information for developing a plan to change the behavior by changing the triggers and consequences. This often involves change on the part of adults, who usually provide the triggers and benefits. BCBAs are trained to make these detailed observations and develop plans for manipulating antecedents and consequences in order to change behavior. Examples of forms used in FBA appear in Appendixes 4A and 4B.

BCBAs and their assistants often are involved in planning and delivering educational programs in which children are taught new, adaptive skills. This aspect of the BCBA's job is discussed in more detail in Chapters 6 and 7.

SPECIAL EDUCATOR/EARLY INTERVENTIONIST

Special education is delivered by teachers who are trained to provide instruction to children with a wide range of disabilities, including those with ASD. Most certified special educators in the United States hold master's degrees from programs accredited by the Council for the Accreditation of Educator Preparation (CAEP; http://caepnet.org). The specialist working with children with disabilities under the age of 3 may be referred to as an early interventionist or an early childhood special educator. The special educator will be part of the team involved in developing the child's individualized family service plan (IFSP) or individualized education program (IEP). (For more information, see Chapter 5 and Appendixes 5A and 5B.) Once the plan is written, the special educator will develop the curriculum and activities to address the goals and objectives listed in the child's plan. These will be delivered by the special educator in collaboration with other team members, who may or may not directly work with the child and family. A large part of the special educator's job is to communicate with parents and coordinate with other team members regarding progress and concerns.

Special educators/early interventionists generally focus on developing the academic and preacademic skills a child will need to benefit from a preschool or school curriculum. These services often are provided in the home for children under 3 years old and are aimed at developing play and self-help skills that will allow children to interact with peers as well as preacademic skills such as language and communication; concepts such as colors, shapes, and numbers; and preliteracy skills such as alphabet knowledge and experience with books and stories. Many of these skills overlap with what the SLP will focus on, and the two will often work in collaboration. The special educator/early interventionist may do the bulk of the direct service, with input from the SLP and other team members as to what aspects of the preacademic curriculum to target and how to facilitate the child's acquisition of important skills and concepts.

Programming usually takes place in a preschool classroom for children who are 3–5 years old. Current law governing special education, the Individuals with Disabilities Education Act of 2004 (IDEA), requires that all children with disabilities be educated with children without disabilities as much as possible and have access to the general education curriculum to as great an extent as possible. This requirement often is referred to as the least restrictive environment (LRE). To fulfill it, a child may be placed in an inclusive preschool setting (placing children with special educational needs in classes with children who have typical development) with support from a special educator, in a reverse mainstream classroom, where most children have special needs but several typically developing peers participate, or in a special education classroom that has some scheduled activities with a group of typically developing peers from another classroom. Placement depends on the child's level of functioning, parental preference, and availability within the local education agency (LEA), which has the responsibility to provide a free appropriate public education (FAPE) for the child.

The ability to participate fully in the general education curriculum is a major determiner for placing school-age children in the appropriate classroom. Those who can fully participate are usually placed in an inclusive classroom with some special education support. Some inclusive classrooms allow for modified curricula to accommodate children with more severe disabilities. These classrooms may contain a combination of children who do and do not have special needs and use a teaching methodology called integrated co-teaching (ICT), which allows a special educator and a general education teacher to collaborate on all areas of the curriculum and work with all students. Alternatively, students with more significant special needs may be placed in an inclusive classroom for certain parts of the day and in a special education classroom for others. Another option is to have a full-time aide who helps the child with special needs take part in aspects of the curriculum while providing tutoring support for areas of instruction that are part of the student's IEP. Therapists including SLPs and OTs often will collaborate with general and special education teachers to create lessons or activities for the student and may work collaboratively within the classroom alongside the general and special educators. Chapter 5 provides more detailed information about the educational services for children with ASD. The special educator working in a classroom will:

- Observe and assess requirements of each child with special needs to increase success in the classroom

- Modify the environment (minimize distractions; auditory or visual)

- Allow extra time for processing of information

- Modify lesson plans (materials, incorporating IEP goals)

- Create a sense of predictability through schedules and visuals of steps for lessons and activities (task analysis)

- Model/coach effective teaching strategies for staff to observe and replicate

- Implement behavioral support plans so that they are consistent among all staff

- Take data on student behavior

- Collaborate with therapists to help create an IEP

- Assist staff and other children in understanding the child's needs

- Make sure there are opportunities for interaction and communication (e.g., peer editing in writing, playing a math game with a partner, turning and talking to a peer on the rug)

- Provide visual supports and monitor peer interactions to make them successful

- Use specific peer coaching strategies, such as a buddy system, to help peers serve as models, motivators, and social initiators for the child with ASD

- Help achieve academic and social IEP goals and create the goals for the following school year

SOCIAL WORKER

The primary mission of the social worker is to help clients meet basic human needs, with particular attention to the needs and empowerment of people who are vulnerable, oppressed, and living in poverty. Social workers focus on individual well-being in a social context and on the well-being of society. They may hold a bachelor's (BSW) or master's degree (MSW) in social work from a program accredited by the Council on Social Work Education (CSWE; http://www.cswe.org). Social workers in early intervention and preschool programs may serve as liaisons between the program and family, coordinate services among the team, and assist the family in obtaining services and resources that they need but are outside the scope of educational agencies. Social workers in a school setting serve as advocates to ensure children are receiving the appropriate educational experiences and help obtain access to other services the family may need, including:

- Family assessments and resources that may include housing and financial assistance

- Assistance with navigation through social services systems

- Helping to coordinate the school's special education team to ensure that children with special needs have a positive educational experience

- Counseling services for children as part of their IEPs; counseling services may also be provided around family issues, social-emotional problems, bullying, and so forth

- Consulting to general education and special education teachers regarding behavioral interventions for children who are difficult in the classroom or around suspicion of possible child abuse or neglect

- Social skills development programs for students with ASD and other social-emotional needs

- Staff development training to ensure inclusive classrooms run smoothly and that general education and special education teachers are fully trained in different methods for accommodating children with special needs

EDUCATIONAL AIDES/PARAPROFESSIONALS

Educational aides/paraprofessionals work with educators and therapists to deliver a program designed by the professional. They may hold a bachelor's degree, but many hold a high school diploma or an associate's degree. They often do not have training in special education and most are trained on the job. These individuals may work in schools or birth-to-3 agencies and provide in-home services to young children. It is imperative that the program they deliver is designed and overseen by a qualified professional special educator or therapist. Parents have a right to know the qualifications of interventionists sent to their homes and to be in touch with the supervising professionals and therapists who need to oversee and evaluate the aide's work.

Many children with ASD who are in preschool and school settings are assigned paraprofessional aides who work individually with them within a classroom setting. This can help the child to focus on tasks, complete work, avoid distractions and off-task behavior, and interact successfully with peers. It is, however, important for parents to understand that an aide is not a program. Aides are only as effective as the program designed and overseen by the professionals whose responsibility it is to create appropriate instruction for the child. The aide can help the child concentrate on and work through the program, and many children with disabilities have close, nurturing relationships with their aides. The aide cannot, however, independently decide what the child needs to learn and do throughout the course of the school day because of his or her limited training and expertise. That is the job of the educational team, which creates the child's educational plan and instructs the aide in implementing it. The aide may, though, participate in the IEP and contribute knowledge about the child's day-to-day behavior.

PHYSICIANS

The physician's role is to identify or rule out medical causes of the child's developmental disability, prescribe and manage medications for symptoms, and consult about issues around basic bodily functions, such as eating, sleeping, and elimination. You may decide or be referred to visit the following physicians, depending on your child's needs.

Child Psychiatrist

In addition to having specialized training in neurodevelopmental disabilities that assists in diagnosis and treatment planning, child psychiatrists manage medications aimed at addressing symptoms of ASD such as anxiety. Although parents are naturally wary of using medications with young children, they are sometimes helpful in alleviating symptoms in a severe condition such as ASD. Consultation with a child psychiatrist can be useful in deciding what, if any, medications might be useful in helping your child reduce unwanted behavior and be more available for learning opportunities.

Developmental Pediatrician

Developmental pediatricians are trained to work with children and their families and have additional training that helps them recognize and participate in the evaluation of children with developmental disabilities, including ASD. Although general pediatricians are qualified to diagnose ASD, a minority of pediatricians have specialized training in child development and disabilities. If your family pediatrician makes the diagnosis of ASD for your child, then you may want to ask for a referral to a developmental specialist.

Whether a developmental specialist or not, your family pediatrician will manage the medications and treatments for the normal childhood illnesses, such as ear infections, rashes, and childhood diseases. The pediatrician will also make sure your child has all the vaccinations necessary to protect from serious childhood illnesses. Although you may have heard some scare stories about dangers of childhood immunizations, a large number of studies from all over the world have now established that there is no link between childhood vaccination and autism (for more information, see Offit & Bell [2003]). All children are safest when fully vaccinated (See Appendix 4C for more detail).

Pediatric Neurologist

The pediatric neurologist may also make a diagnosis of ASD. Most pediatricians recommend that families see a pediatric neurologist when a diagnosis of ASD is made in order to find out whether the ASD is associated with any known (and perhaps treatable) neurological syndrome or disease. In the minority of cases, the appearance of ASD can be traced to a neurological disease such as neurofibromatosis. In addition, seizures sometimes accompany autism, and this aspect of the syndrome may be managed by a neurologist. In most cases, the pediatric neurologist will rule out any identifiable causes or accompanying syndromes. The cause of ASD unfortunately will remain unknown for most children.

Gastroenterologist

Although there is no well-established connection between digestive problems and ASD, many claims about gut–brain connections in ASD have been made. There does appear to be a higher prevalence of certain kinds of digestive problems, primarily constipation and feeding sensitivities, in children with ASD, although most researchers believe these are more related to behavioral than strictly gastroenterological issues (Ibrahim, Voight, Katusic, Weaver, & Barbaresi, 2009; McElhanin, McCracken, Karpen, & Shar, 2014). Many families will seek the aid of a gastroenterologist to identify treatable syndromes that may co-occur with ASD or rule out organic diseases as a source of the child's symptoms. There is no evidence, though, that any treatment for stomach or digestive problems is effective in eliminating core symptoms of ASD.

HOW CAN PARENTS HELP THEIR CHILD'S TEAM COLLABORATE EFFECTIVELY?

The team of professionals who may be involved in your child's educational program can be large. Your role as a parent is to make sure that all the team members understand the "big picture" for your child—the program goals that are a high priority for you, the behavioral strategies being used to minimize maladaptive behavior, and the rewards that are most effective for your child. Although your team will periodically meet as a whole, you can speed up the process of communication by letting one team member know what another is doing and how it is working, passing on successful strategies discovered by other team members, and sharing the methods you've seen team members use that keep maladaptive behavior to a minimum. In addition, team members should be involving you in their individual sessions to make sure you can carry over the techniques they find successful and can share them with others on the team. You are the connection between your child and the many members of the team, so you play a pivotal role in keeping the communication among the team going.

Example Functional
Behavior Analysis (FBA) Form

TARGET BEHAVIOR: _____

ACTIVITY: _____

DATE/TIME:

Setting events	Antecedents	Behavior	Consequences
What sets the stage for problem behavior?	*What immediate triggers precede problem behavior?*	*What does the problem behavior look like?*	*What immediately follows problem behavior?*
❑ Lack of sleep ❑ Meds side effects ❑ Illness or pain ❑ Chronic medical condition ❑ Fatigue ❑ Hunger/thirst ❑ Fight/conflict with peers ❑ Recently reprimanded ❑ Teased or bullied ❑ Anxious, agitated ❑ Overstimulating/noisy environment ❑ Activity long, boring, disliked ❑ Conflict in the home/bus/cafeteria ❑ Having to wait for a long time ❑ Setting event not known ❑ Other (specify)	❑ Changed routine or schedule ❑ Ended or interrupted activity ❑ Making a transition ❑ Denied access/removal of preferred activity ❑ Told "No, Don't, Stop" ❑ Asked to wait ❑ Presence or absence of a certain person ❑ Reduced level of attention provided ❑ Unable to complete a task/activity ❑ Told or asked to do something ❑ Made a mistake or was corrected ❑ Given unclear expectations/directions ❑ Sudden/unexpected event (e.g., loud noise) ❑ Trigger not known ❑ Other (specify)	❑ Noncompliance ❑ Aggression towards others ❑ Verbal refusal ❑ Disruptions ❑ Crying ❑ Screaming/yelling ❑ Kicking/hitting ❑ Running away/bolting ❑ Destroying property ❑ Making verbal threats ❑ Other (specify)	❑ Given teacher attention (e.g., redirection, correction, warnings) ❑ Given peer attention (e.g., laughing, negative reaction) ❑ Given assistance or help ❑ Behavior ignored (i.e., attention withdrawn) ❑ Given access to an object/activity ❑ Request or demand withdrawn ❑ Request or demand delayed ❑ Avoids tasks, activity, or situation ❑ Removed from activity/area ❑ Removed object or preferred item ❑ Other (specify)
Notes:	Notes:	Intensity: *Low/Medium/High* Duration in minutes 1–5/5–10/10–30	Notes:

Sources: O'Neill, Horner, Albin, Sprague, Storey, & Newton (1997); Dunlap, Iovannone, English, Kincaid, Wilson, Christiansen, & Strain (2010). Adapted by permission from Bleiweiss, J., Hough, L., & Cohen, S. (2013). *Everyday classroom strategies and practices for supporting children with autism spectrum disorders.* Shawnee Mission, KS: Autism Asperger Publishing Company.

Setting Events-Antecedent-Behavior-Consequence Chart (SABC)

Setting Events-Antecedent-Behavior-Consequence Chart (Bleiweiss, 2010)

Please fill out the following data chart as soon as possible following any disruptive or interfering behavior displayed. The information you provided for each section of the table will help create a comprehensive picture of the circumstances triggering and maintaining the targeted behavior.

STUDENT'S NAME: _____   TARGET BEHAVIOR: _____

Context (Briefly describe the line, activity, nature, and place of the activity or task)	Setting events (Describe biological, environmental, social and factors that may contribute to the behavior)	Antecedent (what immediately precedes the behavior?)	Behavior (Measurable observable terms; frequency, duration, intensity)	Consequences (Response/reaction to the behavior; what happened afterwards)
Date: **Time:** **Activity/task:**				
Date: **Time:** **Activity/task:**				
Date: **Time:** **Activity/task:**				

From Bleiweiss, J.D. (2013). Using a positive behavior support framework in the ASD nest classroom. In S. Cohen & L. Hough (Eds.), *The ASD nest model: An inclusion program for students with autism spectrum disorders* (pp. 81–93). Shawnee Mission, KS: Autism Asperger Publishing Company.

Parents Ask

Am I Risking Autism If I Vaccinate My Children?

There is no evidence that autism is caused by any vaccine or any additive or preservative ever used in one. There have been large, well-controlled studies done all over the Western world that have confirmed this finding over and over again. There is no reason for any parent to deny a child the crucial protection today's vaccines offer out of misguided fear that doing so would increase the risk for autism. Although science can never absolutely prove that something will not happen—we can't be absolutely 100% sure that it will never snow on Jan. 1 in Kinsangani in the equatorial Congo, for instance—science can reassure us that the likelihood of certain events is vanishingly small. But apart from thinking about how tiny the risk of an action like providing children with vaccinations might be, we also need to think about the risk of taking the opposite action. What are the risks of NOT vaccinating your children?

Most parents of children today never experienced any of the classic childhood diseases because they themselves were vaccinated. But I am old enough to remember when things were different. Although I did receive some of the first polio vaccines, immunizations for the other then common childhood diseases were not available when I was a kid. Let me tell you about these diseases. Between the time I was about 4 and 7, I contracted measles, mumps, what we then called German measles or rubella, what we called whooping cough or pertussis, chicken pox, and scarlet fever. So did my younger brother and sister, but I always seemed to get the most severe case. When I got chicken pox I developed severe scarring, particularly on my forehead, and for my whole life I have always felt I had to wear my hair in a certain way to hide the scars. If you have never seen a child with whooping cough, I hope you never have to, because even though I was only four when I had it, I still remember how painful that cough was, and how scary it was to feel I couldn't breathe. I can hardly imagine what my parents must have felt hearing me cough and gasp for breath like that for weeks on end. My parents were shopkeepers. They had no employees; they ran their store together and when we kids were sick, my father had to run it alone. Although my brother and sister usually recovered in a week or two, I was down for weeks with each infection. As a complication of one of these bouts, I developed rheumatic fever. I was hospitalized, then when I developed heart complications, transferred from our local hospital to Children's in Philadelphia, 3 hours from my home. With a toddler and an infant at home and a store to run, my parents weren't at the hospital much. I was five, and I can still see myself in that hospital bed; still feel the fierce loneliness I experienced during my time there. I developed a chronic heart murmur. I wasn't allowed to participate in any sports or vigorous activities during my childhood. The murmur had to be monitored during each of my children's births. I still have to take antibiotics whenever I have any kind of potential bleeding, even in a procedure as simple as a dental cleaning. Given the choice, I would never have opted to risk that my own children would suffer as I did. I'm deeply grateful that I was able protect them from these illnesses.

But really, I was lucky. My complications were relatively limited. Anyone who has seen the movie *The Miracle Worker* knows that Helen Keller was a precocious 18 month

With kind permission from Springer Science+Business Media: From Paul, R. (2009). Ask the experts: Am I risking autism if I vaccinate my children? *Journal of Autism and Developmental Disorders, 39*(6), 962–963.

old who had already started to talk when she was struck with measles, which was accompanied by encephalitis, leaving her blind and deaf for life. In the 1960s there was an epidemic of rubella, which infected pregnant women, causing damage to their not-yet-born children. There is a cohort of people who are now adults living with severe disabilities—deafness, blindness, and mental retardation—as a result of this epidemic. And children die from these diseases, too. They didn't in Western countries for quite a while because immunization was virtually universal. But they did before the advent of vaccines, and they are again now that parents are abstaining from them. Seven unvaccinated children died last year in the UK from these diseases.

If we were to compare risks mathematically, the risk of death or disability as a result of not vaccinating a child, while small, is significantly larger than the (probably near zero) risk of causing an autism spectrum disorder by immunizing. Some parents may say, "I don't care how small the risk is, I don't want to take it with my child." But the truth is if you refuse to take one immensely small risk, you are exposing your child to a much larger one; the risk of contracting and suffering severe complications of a disease from which protection is readily, cheaply, and almost painlessly available. Maybe you have heard that the reason the "establishment" is in favor of vaccination is because it makes money for the drug companies.

Maybe you've been told there is a conspiracy to suppress the risks of vaccination to keep money flowing to the pharmaceutical houses and their stock holders; or that government officials worked with drug firms to keep risks quiet because they were "on the take." Although drug companies do make some money from vaccines, no one has ever been able to establish that there has been financial malfeasance of any kind among supporters of vaccination. In fact, the opposite is true. Dr. Paul Offit has shown how many of the most vocal vaccine critics are in league with, and receive funds from lawyers who want to get big settlements from drug companies and the government by suing for alleged damage to children.

We live in complex times; yes, there are many difficult choices and real risks that parents need to weigh in making sure our children grow up safe, healthy, and prepared for the demands of this fast-changing world. But deciding whether or not to vaccinate is not one of these difficult choices. The benefits are clear and inarguable. The risks are miniscule. On the other hand, the risks of not vaccinating are sizable and getting larger. As more people refuse vaccination, these diseases have increased opportunities to take hold, spread, and infect a larger proportion of the unprotected. Vaccines for childhood illnesses are a blessing we ought to celebrate. Not only do they save lives and protect against serious disability, they reduce suffering for children and their families, who won't have to face as many challenges as my parents did in dealing with children who are very sick for a lot of their childhood. This argument ought to be long over. There are so many more pressing needs for children with autism and their families to confront. We ought to work together to overcome those, and not waste any more time and treasure on this dead horse.

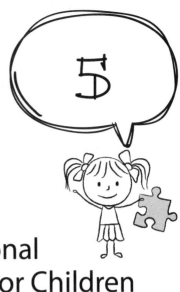

What Types of Educational Services Are Available for Children with Autism Spectrum Disorder?

The process of getting a diagnosis and arranging the services your child needs can be overwhelming and stressful. In addition, you have probably already met several well-intentioned professionals who may be throwing around words, phrases, and abbreviations that sound like a foreign language to you (see Box 5.1 for a list of terms used by professionals). It's natural to be confused about what all these new terms mean. It may not be easy to get all the information you need on the services your child can gain access to at different points in development. Chapter 4 talked about the professionals likely to have a role in your child's intervention and education. This section focuses on some of the terms these professionals are likely to use, and the chapter introduces you to the range of services that are available throughout childhood and beyond. The chapter also provides you with a road map and vocabulary to help navigate the world of both special education and the other services that may be available for your child. Guidelines for gathering information for the most appropriate education program also are provided, and there is a discussion regarding sources of insurance coverage for services. Let's start with services provided under the umbrella of special education.

Educational Terms Used by Professionals

The Arc   The Arc of the United States; One of the largest national community-based advocacy groups for people with intellectual and developmental disabilities and their families

AAC   Augmentative and alternative communication

EA   Educational aid

EEN   Exceptional educational need

FAPE   Free appropriate public education

IDEA (Part B and Part C)   Individuals with Disabilities Education Improvement Act of 2004 (PL 108-446)

IEP   Individualized education program

IFSP   Individualized family service plan

inclusion   Supporting students with disabilities in general education and community settings to access mainstream activities and education with necessary supports provided by educators and therapists.

LEA   Local education agency

LRE   Least restrictive environment; an educational setting that allows your child to have the most contact possible within an educational setting with children without disabilities and access to the general education curriculum

mainstreaming   Including children with disabilities in general education classrooms

NCLB   No Child Left Behind Act of 2001 (PL 107-110)

paraprofessional/para   Individual working under the direction of a professional teacher or therapist

peer models   Typically developing children who work or play along with children with disabilities in educational programs

related services   Instruction or therapy provided by individuals other than teachers (e.g., Speech Language Pathologists, Occupational Therapists) for students with disabilities

reverse mainstream   Classroom including students with disabilities along with peer models

services and supports   The help provided to students with disabilities within an educational program, including services of therapists, paraprofessionals, and special education teachers, as well as environmental help such as visual schedules and AAC devices

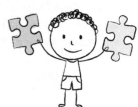

SEIT   Special education itinerant teacher

SSA   Social Security Administration

SSDI   Social Security Disability Insurance

SSI   Supplemental Security Income

SEN   Special educational needs

WHAT IS SPECIAL EDUCATION?

Special education refers to instruction designed to meet the individual needs of children with disabilities. Federal mandates in the United States dictate the services that children in need of special education are legally entitled to receive. The way these services are delivered can vary greatly, however, depending on where you live. Some states label the recipients of these services as having *special educational needs* and others will use the term *exceptional educational needs*. Students in special education also may be referred to as students who are "on IEPs." What's important to know is that all of these terms refer to children with disabilities who are entitled to services through IDEA 2004. Special education is provided by professionals who are trained to work with children with different kinds of learning issues, sometimes referred to as *exceptionalities*; these educators can assess students' needs, provide the appropriate teaching methods to enable learning, and work with general education teachers to make accommodations for the child within the classroom. Special education professionals may be assisted by aides, but IDEA requires that professional educators and therapists manage assessment and treatment planning and supervise the work of paraprofessionals.

Federal mandates in the United States dictate the services that children in need of special education are legally entitled to receive. The way these services are delivered can vary greatly, however, depending on where you live.

Children gain access to special education through referral and assessment. Referrals can come from parents or educators; anyone concerned about a child's performance can initiate a referral for an assessment of special educational need. Parents always have the option whether to consent to an assessment, but they don't have to initiate the process themselves. If a teacher notices a problem that has not been identified before, then a request to obtain parental permission for an assessment can be made.

Most children with ASD will have already had these referrals made before they get to public school, often through birth-to-3 systems. Some children, particularly those with high verbal abilities, may not be recognized as having a disability until they get to school, though. In these cases, referral and assessment for special educational need may happen when the child starts a school program.

Children ages 3–21 are mandated by IDEA to receive a free appropriate public education, abbreviated as FAPE. This usually means that after an assessment demonstrates that the child meets criteria for eligibility for special education, parents and educators get together to decide what form the special services will take. In most cases, this will mean supports for the child, including provision of therapies such as speech-language; occupational, physical, and behavior therapy; extra help for the teacher and child in the form of an educational aide; and perhaps placement in a specialized classroom for all or part of the school day. If the LEA does not believe they can provide an adequate program for the child, then they may recommend a specialized day or residential program outside the local district. Parents and educators will document their decision in an IEP once consensus about the types and intensity of support is reached at a meeting designed to develop the educational plan for the child.

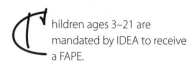 hildren ages 3–21 are mandated by IDEA to receive a FAPE.

Most families are able to find common ground with their educational team and can agree on the content of the child's FAPE. Families occasionally find that LEAs are unable or unwilling to provide the kinds of special services the family believes are best for the child. We'll talk a little later about what might happen when this is the case.

If IDEA Mandates a Free Appropriate Public Education Only for Children Ages 3–21, Will We Have to Pay for Services Before Our Child Is 3 Years Old?

Early intervention services are those provided to children with special needs before the age of 3. Some children, such as those with Down syndrome or congenital deafness, begin early intervention when they are infants because their disabilities can be identified at birth. Children with ASD, however, usually cannot be diagnosed until later in development, so their services typically begin later. Part C of IDEA is a federal grant program that assists states in developing and operating statewide programs of early intervention services for infants and toddlers with disabilities. As of this writing, all states and U.S. territories are participating in the Part C program. The law requires that states provide assessment of eligibility for early intervention services free of charge, but once a child is identified as needing services, states do not have to provide them for free. Some states do have free early intervention programs but others require families to pay for the services on a sliding scale. To find out about services in your state, search for "birth to three" and your state's name.

Birth-to-3 services are designed to be family-centered, which means that the family plays a central role in making decisions about assessment and intervention programs and procedures. The family is considered the foundation for supporting skill development

he family is considered the foundation for supporting skill development and learning for children younger than age 3.

and learning for children younger than age 3. Let's look at what Part C services might be like through the eyes of Niko and his family.

Niko's parents became concerned when he still wasn't talking by 2 years of age. Their pediatrician referred them to the local birth-to-3 agency, which carried out a comprehensive assessment. Following the evaluation, Niko's parents met with a team of professionals who had expertise in ASD. The team observed and evaluated Niko and concluded that he exhibited significant developmental delay with symptoms of ASD. Niko was deemed eligible for early intervention services and qualified for Part C services under IDEA. Niko's parents experienced mixed feelings as they listened to the team report their findings. They were relieved to hear that Niko would be eligible to receive home-based intervention and that they would be involved in setting goals for their son, but they were heartbroken to learn that their son had a serious, chronic disability. At the same time, they felt that the team was seeing Niko clearly and worked with them to develop a set of goals for therapy that they felt were most important for Niko's development. Although the therapists thought Niko might not be ready to start talking and should work first on nonverbal communication, the SLP took the parents' desire for Niko to begin speaking into account and included work on vocal communication in his service plan. Although Niko's parents were initially uneasy about teaching a child as young as Niko, the family became comfortable with the team of service providers over time and came to feel they showed skill and sensitivity in working with Niko in ways that seemed appropriate for his age.

The SLP worked directly with Niko once a week on communication skills, understanding language, and using sounds. The SLP also met weekly with the rest of the team to talk about how to incorporate her communication goals into occupational therapy and special education sessions, which Niko received twice a week from the OT and three times a week from the early intervention specialist.

Niko showed progress between his second and third birthday. He began using a few words, including *mama,* which made his mother very happy. He learned to feed himself with a spoon, and he began stacking blocks instead of sniffing or throwing them. His posture also improved and it was easier for him to sit for a bath. But his parents were still worried. What would happen after Niko turned 3 years old? Would he still receive services, and would the same team work with him, or would they have to start this process all over again? The intervention team began to discuss this transition with the family several months before Niko's third birthday. The team informed Niko's parents about the programs available in their school district, encouraged them to visit each program, and prompted them to be ready to discuss how to manage the transition at the next team meeting. Niko's parents felt better knowing that their son's services would continue and that their views about the best program for Niko would be respected and taken into consideration during transition planning.

A partnership between parents and professionals is essential in the early years. The goal of IDEA Part C is to provide coordinated services for children from birth to 3 years who have identified disabilities such as Niko. That's why an IFSP is used as a service planning document for children under 3. The IFSP documents the decisions made by the family and team about

- Short- and long-term goals that the family and professionals have identified as areas that need intervention

- The treatment methods to be used

- Recommendations for the family to help them participate in the child's development

- Progress monitoring and assessment methods

- The location of intervention services

- A transition plan to school-based services at age 3

The IFSP includes the needs and priorities identified by the family and encourages parental participation in all stages of planning, treatment, and transition (see Appendix 5A for a sample example of IFSP content).

What Happens When Our Child Who Is Receiving Early Intervention Turns 3 Years Old?

Part B of IDEA covers services for children ages 3–21 and requires that these services be provided as part of FAPE in a school setting, including preschool for children ages 3–5. Children over the age of 3 are no longer eligible for Part C services and make the transition into the public school system. This can be a stressful time for families of children with ASD because it may involve services outside the home for the first time and it requires getting to know a new team of educators and service providers. In addition, parents may feel less in touch with their child's program when services move to a school setting. Transitional planning services are built into IDEA Part C to avoid these kinds of stressors. IFSPs must begin to address transition to school before the child's third birthday, and families are encouraged to start working with their LEA before that milestone. There is a lot of responsibility placed on parents in a family-centered program to coordinate and monitor their child's services. It can be helpful during this time to reach out to parent support groups as well as individuals in your area who have already navigated the school transition process. You may also want to utilize online resources to identify local service options and visit the programs for which your child is a candidate.

The IFSP is replaced with an IEP once a child makes the transition to the public school system. The IEP lists the child's educational goals and must be approved by the parents, who must be included in the IEP planning process. The IEP differs from the IFSP in a number of ways. Most important, the IEP focus shifts to the child in the educational setting rather than the child in the family setting. Children with ASD may continue to have challenges and needs at home even though services are now primarily confined to the school. If this is the case, then parents have the right to request services that they consider essential for school readiness. For example, you may request support at home for maladaptive behaviors that are dangerous (e.g., self-injury, inability to sleep at night) or interfere with the process of generalizing school learning to other settings. In addition, parents might request an alternative augmentative communication device such as an iPad or other communication aid at home if one is being used for communication at school. Many students with ASD have difficulty using verbal language and may be unable to practice communication skills learned at school in the home environment or convey information from school to home. Parents can request a two-way communication system so parents can be informed of daily activities and also have the opportunity to communicate concerns or celebrate progress. This is usually a written log that goes back and forth between the school and the home.

What Are Preschool Services Like for Children with ASD?

Education for children ages 3–5 with special needs usually takes place in a preschool classroom. One goal of IDEA is to have children with disabilities educated in the LRE. LRE is usually interpreted to mean 1) in the neighborhood school, if possible, or in one as close to it as possible and 2) in a general education classroom (sometimes called a *mainstream* or *inclusion* class), if possible, and with at least some opportunity to interact with typically developing peers (see Chapter 4). What is possible is usually determined by 1) a child's ability to participate in and benefit from the general curriculum and 2) the child's own safety and that of others when functioning in a typical classroom (see Chapter 4). The IEP will specify the type of preschool setting that the parents and educational team both agree is most appropriate for the child.

Barriers for preschool children to participate in a regular class are somewhat lower than at the grade school level. A significant portion of the preschool curriculum focuses on play, communication, and social interaction, which benefit all children in a preschool classroom, both with and without disabilities. Preschoolers with ASD usually have a range of options in the classroom as long as children with ASD and their classmates are safe and comfortable in the shared classroom environment (i.e., children do not exhibit behaviors that would make the setting dangerous). Several kinds of programs may be offered to a child with ASD, depending on level of functioning:

- *An inclusive preschool class:* Children take part in a typical preschool in this setting. Mainstream, or inclusive, classrooms are placed within a grade school or housed in community preschools that work with the LEA to provide "slots" for students in special education. Your child may receive support from any of the professionals discussed in Chapter 4, including a special educator, paraprofessional (sometimes called a "para" or an educational aide), or special education teacher, as part of the placement. A paraprofessional may be assigned to either an individual child or to a classroom to provide the extra help needed. Therapists, including SLPs, OTs, and PTs, may work with your child in the classroom or in a separate area during the school day.

- *A reverse mainstream classroom:* Most children in this type of classroom have special needs of some kind. Several preschoolers with typical development also participate as peer models. The primary teacher may be a general or special educator. Reverse mainstream classrooms typically have more than one aide to assist the teacher, and therapists work with individuals or small groups within or outside the classroom during the school day. Each child with special needs has an IEP, and the curriculum targets goals shared among the students with special needs. IEP targets that are less common may be taught to individuals or small groups by therapists; these targets will be practiced in activities provided by the aides and overseen by the therapists.

- *A special education classroom:* These classrooms are similar to the reverse mainstream set-up. Each child with special needs has scheduled activities with a group of typically developing peers from another class within the school building instead of having peer models enrolled in the same class as the child with special needs. The pairings are determined by child needs, level of functioning, parental preference, and availability. The primary teacher for this class is likely to be a special educator, although in some districts SLPs take this role. The special education classroom will probably have several aides to assist the teacher, and therapists will visit to work with individuals or small groups inside or outside the classroom. Aides or therapists may accompany children when they visit their peers' classrooms to coach interactions and reinforce play and social skills targeted in IEPs.

How Does the Individualized Education Plan Work to Organize Services for My Child at School Age?

The IEP documents educational goals, the services that will be provided, and the location of each special service (e.g., an inclusive classroom or special education classroom within the neighborhood school or other local school, a separate location such as a therapy room within the home, school, or special school). In addition to documenting where each service the child receives will take place, the IEP also describes how the goals will be measured and the date of the next review meeting. The IEP is typically updated annually at a meeting with parents and the school team. Children are reassessed, with parental consent, toward the end of the year when the IEP is due for renewal. The special education team, which includes the parents and related services providers (e.g., SLP, OT, social worker), then meets to discuss the child's progress in relation to the goals listed in the IEP. The team also will discuss concerns and make recommendations for the upcoming new IEP.

The annual meeting is a good time to review progress, see how far your child has progressed, and look at what is working well in the program and what needs to be changed or reevaluated. For example, if the team decides the child needs additional accommodations, such as a voice output communication device to "speak," then these changes are documented in the IEP. Jessa's case is an example of how this might work. (See Appendix 5B for a sample IEP.)

Jessa's OT, Ms. Barton, reported at the IEP meeting that she had been working on hand skills, such as holding a crayon or pencil, in her therapy room outside of Jessa's primary special education class to help Jessa learn to write her name. (This type of service is often referred to as *pull-out.*) Jessa's parents, Liz and Gary, talked at the annual IEP

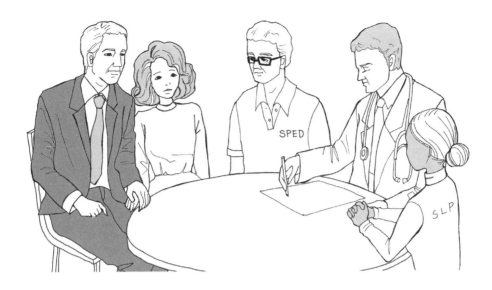

meeting about how pleased they were that Jessa was writing her name and said she was showing interest in writing other things, often spending time after school writing at home and playing with the magnetic letters they kept on the refrigerator. They also talked about how eager they were for Jessa to spend more time in the inclusive first grade. Ms. Barton suggested that she could spend some of her time with Jessa working in the first-grade classroom during handwriting time, and she could work with Jessa and some of the other first graders who were having trouble with writing to practice writing the words the first graders are working on for sight word reading. (Therapy that takes place in the classroom often is called *push-in service,* although the more correct term is *collaborative service*.) The team agreed to move Jessa's OT services from pull-out to collaborative in the first-grade classroom. Her IEP was modified to specify the location of OT services from a separate location to a general education classroom.

It is especially important that parents of children with ASD discuss not only academics with the child's intervention team but also social skills, language and communication, functional skills, and ADLs. Growth in these areas increases children's chances for success in the general curriculum as well as at home and in community life outside of the school, and the services to support them belong on the IEP. The aim of special education is for each child to reach his or her maximum potential and be able to lead the most independent life possible. Social and adaptive skills contribute to this aim in crucial ways. For some children with ASD who are attending inclusive classrooms in public schools, in fact, it may not be the academic skills that hold them back. Some students with ASD are quite competent academically. They usually struggle, however, to communicate and interact with adults and peers. This social difficulty tends to impede classroom learning, hinder the development of independence, and cause frustration and loneliness. In order to provide an appropriate program that enables children with

ASD to succeed within the general curriculum and develop toward independent living,
as the law requires, these programs will need
to address social communication and activities of daily living as well as the three Rs (reading, writing, arithmetic), and these additional
goals should be documented on the IEP.

I t is especially important that
parents of children with ASD
discuss not only academics
with the child's intervention team
but also social skills, language and
communication, functional skills,
and activities of daily living.

Will Our Child with ASD Have to Be in a "Special Class" When He or She Gets to School?

Although there often are opportunities for preschool and kindergarten children
with ASD to participate in inclusive preschool settings that combine children
with and without disabilities, some LEAs offer limited options for children with
special needs once they enter the primary grades. Parents may be distressed to
find that their school team recommends a special classroom placement for a
school-age child with ASD who has been functioning in an inclusive preschool
or kindergarten. This may happen because the school team does not think
the child with ASD will be able to master the general curriculum of the classroom, such as learning to read and doing basic math. Parents in this situation
often feel frightened that their child will fall behind without the expectations
of the general curriculum and their child may become isolated and develop
less adaptive behavior without the peer models of the general classroom. This
recommendation is usually made when it is suspected that the student will
do better in a smaller classroom with more support and more opportunity for
individualized instruction.

Children with strong verbal skills often can benefit from the challenge of
the curriculum in the inclusive classroom, but they may have difficulties with its
complex rules, levels of noise and activity, and busy social scene. There may be
some advantage for some of these children to spending at least part of the school
day in a smaller group in which there is more opportunity for individual attention. Children with lower cognitive and language skills may also benefit from the
social opportunities of the inclusive class, even if they need to have a curriculum
designed for them with limited participation in the subject matter of the rest of
the class. But they, too, may find a smaller, quieter, more individualized environment to be more conducive to learning, at least some of the time. There is never
just one right answer that works for every child, even though there are trends in
education that favor inclusion.

IDEA 2004 was closely aligned to the No Child Left Behind Act (NCLB) of
2001 (PL 107-110). Using evidence-based practices to enhance progress in the curriculum for all students was one focus of NCLB. Educators have an obligation to
work toward achieving some of the goals of the general curriculum (e.g., learning to read, to write, and do math) for every single child, regardless of what classroom a child attends. Inclusive placements may be effective for accomplishing

these goals for some children if they provide all specialized services (e.g., work with therapists, resources for teachers and special educators to collaborate to implement IEP and appropriate curriculum modifications) and supports (e.g., extra time, individual attention, assistive devices when appropriate) necessary. However, a special education classroom can also address these goals. Whether children are placed in an inclusive classrooms or not their teachers have the responsibility to make sure they attain the goals of the general curriculum.

ICT is one service model that provides a middle road between fully inclusive and special education. ICT involves two teachers who are both responsible for the group of students in their shared classroom; ICT classrooms usually include one teacher certified in general education and another certified in special education. Some ICT classrooms place a general education teacher alongside an SLP. The second teacher may be present only at certain times, and there may be several guest teachers who visit the classroom for particular curricular areas. For example, the reading teacher may assist with literacy instruction for the whole class while children with special education needs receive instruction from the special education teacher. The SLP may work on preliteracy, language comprehension, or social skills, focusing on small groups of children with IEPs, while the general education teacher works with other students on related subjects.

ICT classrooms also may have one or more paraprofessionals to assist the primary teacher. If this is the case, then specific classroom personnel requirements would be indicated in the child's IEP. Paraprofessionals are uncertified personnel who work under the supervision of a certified teacher or therapist. Although most paras are very dedicated and conscientious, they do not have the same level of background knowledge, training, and experience as certified teachers. As we said in Chapter 4, paraprofessionals cannot independently plan or carry out a student's IEP program and must work under the supervision of a professional. They can provide the one-to-one support that a child with ASD may need to manage in a sometimes distracting and highly stimulating classroom. An ICT placement may be a viable option to consider when full inclusion seems difficult to achieve.

It is hard for many parents to accept that their child's primary school placement is in a special education class, and many families believe that their child will have the opportunity to achieve an optimal outcome only in the inclusive classroom. Some states also subscribe to a full inclusion policy for all students with disabilities. If appropriate services and supports are available—including adequately trained and supervised paraprofessionals, collaborative teaching to individualize instruction, consultative services to teachers from clinicians and therapists with time for team consultations built into the school day—then full inclusion classrooms can be successful settings for children with ASD. Full inclusion may not always be the best option for every child, though, particularly if intensive supports are not carefully structured within the inclusive setting. Placing a child in an inclusive classroom will not in itself guarantee an optimal outcome. Successful inclusion requires careful planning and a coordinated team of professionals and paraprofessionals who have the time and resources to make the classroom work for all its students.

You may feel disappointed if your school-age child has been recommended for placement in a special education classroom rather than an inclusive setting, but every child still has the right to be educated along with typically developing peers, even if he or she is placed in a special education class. The inclusive segment of the educational program may take place for only part of the day, whereas at other times the child receives the kind of individualized, focused, and distraction-free instruction needed in order to learn. Your child will still have access to an IEP and all the services it can provide. The IEP will still include academic goals, but there also will be a focus on achieving functional skills that lead to independence, such as functional reading, grooming, or exercising for physical fitness. As children grow into their teenage years, the IEP will begin to focus on transition plans for moving out of the school setting. Individual Transition Plans address vocational training or higher education options as well as employment, community living, and recreation opportunities.

What Happens When Our Child Turns 22 Years Old?

IDEA provides services for students who are 3–21 years old, or until they graduate from high school. Some students with ASD and other disabilities are not able to meet high school graduate requirements, so they may be eligible for transition programs designed to help students who are 18–21 years old make their way from school to the community. Many 18–21 transition programs are housed on college campuses, so the students get a chance to interact with typically developing peers in the gym, cafeteria, and library, as they did in public school. The curriculum for these programs usually involves teaching functional skills such as shopping, taking public transportation, and cooking. It also includes some form of vocational training, such as working with a coach who helps the student master the requirements of a job in the community, and learning to take part in other community activities such as recreation and volunteer work. Teaching students to speak up for themselves and ask for what they need to successfully participate in the life of their communities is another important part of transition programming.

Some students with ASD will be able to complete the high school graduation requirements and go on to a 2- or 4-year college or vocational program. Although they are not entitled to publicly funded services once they graduate, many 2- and 4-year schools now have programs that provide support to students with autism and other disabilities to allow them to function in a college setting. These programs may help with accommodations they need in the classroom, such as extra time for taking tests or special seating, and they may also provide a student with a peer mentor to coach the student with ASD in social situations. Although some colleges provide these services as part of tuition, others may charge additional fees to support students with ASD.

The hardest part of college for many students with ASD isn't the courses, it's the dorm. Life away from home can be hard for a lot of students, but those with ASD may have particular trouble abiding by the written and unwritten rules of dorm life, understanding the needs of their neighbors, and managing the emotions of growing up. Many families of college students with ASD decide that it is better to have the student live at home and attend classes at a local college rather than traveling far away and living on campus.

> The hardest part of college for many students with ASD isn't the courses, it's the dorm.

The public resources available to support life in the community for people with ASD unfortunately can be limited for both high school graduates and non-graduates older than 22 years of age. This picture is changing, though, because of increased awareness about ASD among the general public and the hard work of advocacy done by many families of these children. Some states have begun providing services specifically designed for adults with ASD, as they do for adults with intellectual and physical disabilities. Researchers and practitioners are beginning to develop programs to effectively address the difficulties these individuals face in building independent and satisfying lives. Some examples can be seen at

https://www.autismspeaks.org/audience/adults.

The number and quality of these programs is bound to grow over the next decades, just as evidence-based services for school-age children with ASD has expanded tremendously since the mid-1980s. A range of useful options to support the self-sufficiency and community integration of citizens with ASD will likely be available by the time your young child with ASD grows up.

What If There Is a Disagreement About the Best Placement for Our Child?

Although LEAs usually make sincere efforts to work with families to come to an agreement about what is best for their child, there are times when consensus is very difficult to reach. Parents may have identified a school in another district or a private school that they feel is perfect for their child, whereas the LEA maintains they can create an appropriate program within their own system. It is important for families to understand that court cases aimed at determining what FAPE means in practice have decided that it does not mean the best possible program available, only an appropriate one. If you find a program outside your school district that you think is the best place for your child, then your school may decline to pay for the program if there is a program in place that the district considers appropriate. No educational placement can be made by the school system without your consent, and you, of course, have the option to send your child to any program of your choice. The problem is that your school district may not be obliged to pay for it, and programs for children with disabilities can be extremely expensive. You have the right to challenge a placement that your school offers, and some parents opt to go to court to do so. Sometimes parents prevail and the school district is directed to fund the program parents choose, but this is not always the case. The following is a real-life example (Wright & Wright, 2007).

The parents of Jacob W., a 6-year-old with ASD, met with school officials in 2003 to decide how to make the transition from preschool to kindergarten. The school district proposed an IEP that would place Jacob in kindergarten at a local elementary school. Jacob's parents were dissatisfied with this proposal, believing the local school was not designed to meet Jacob's special needs. They filed a request for an administrative hearing to challenge the school district's proposed IEP.

At the same time, the parents and school district disagreed about which school should be designated as Jacob's "stay-put" placement—the school that Jacob would attend until the administrative hearing and any subsequent appeals took place. A hearing that summer found in favor of the school district—the local school was an adequate placement. The hearing officer urged the parties to work collaboratively toward an acceptable compromise, but Jacob's parents refused and enrolled him in a private school they had chosen.

Subsequent appeals, going up through the courts to the U.S. Court of Appeals and lasting for more than 3 years, eventually came to the same conclusion as the original hearing. Parents were obliged to pay for the cost of Jacob's education at the private school.

Let us venture to offer some advice on this score. Your child is likely to be involved with the public school system until 18 or 21 years of age. That's a long time. You don't want to spend all those years feeling angry and bitter toward the people who are working with your child. Although your school system worries about budget issues, most of the people who work directly with children really do want to do their best. If you believe that the program options offered by your LEA are not offering the approach you prefer, then talk to other parents in the district to learn if there are more options from which to choose. Visit as many schools as you can and see how the classrooms feel. If you don't think the staff of the available programs are adequately trained in ASD, then request additional training for them (such training might be conducted by staff of a program outside your school district that you think does a good job). If you don't find the behavior management adequate, then you can request a consultation from behavior specialists. If you feel the children in the district's special education preschools are at a much different level of functioning than your child, then you can request peer mentors in the classroom or additional hours of peer interaction in an inclusive class.

No program is perfect, and autism is extremely difficult to treat—no one can give you a guaranteed outcome. It's true that the earlier high-quality intervention starts, the better the chance of making a big difference in your child's prognosis, but as long as your child is learning new skills and developing new adaptive behaviors, the exact pace of growth is not definitive, and even the best program can't ensure that your child will make the progress you hope for.

If conflicts arise, you might agree to a trial period, during which you and the school team carefully document progress, before you decide whether a program fits your child. You might consider agreeing to review your child's IEP in 6 months, perhaps with the help of an independent evaluator who specializes in ASD from the education or psychology department of a local university or from the psychiatry or neurology department of a research hospital. Use observation and data collected in the school program to decide whether growth is taking place.

You will need all of your financial and emotional resources for the long haul; it's wise to conserve these resources and fully explore how far you can collaborate with your LEA to craft an appropriate program that your family feels good about. Work collaboratively with your school system to attempt to find consensus. The Suggested Resources section provides some information to help you understand the issues in education for students with disabilities.

What Resources Are Available Outside the Educational System?

For children under 21, publicly funded services must be provided to address special educational needs through birth-to-3 systems and the LEA. Most of these programs will attempt to provide services within their current program options. There are, however, a few other potential sources of financial assistance to supplement the local educational system, which we'll summarize below.

Insurance Coverage for Services It is an unfortunate reality in the United States that having a child with a disability such as ASD can create a financial burden for families. A few states have taken steps to lessen the burden on families by passing insurance reform laws that prohibit the exclusion of children with disabilities from receiving coverage for services. Such laws vary state by state and depend on your insurance carrier and policy type. Families can check with the office of the state insurance commissioner (see http://www.naic.org/state_web _map.htm for help finding the office in your state) or local office of advocacy organizations such as Family Voices (a national network to provide families with resources and support to make informed decisions, advocate for improved public and private policies, build partnerships among families and professionals, and serve as a resource on health care; http://www.familyvoices.org), The Arc of the United States (The Arc; one of the largest national community-based advocacy groups for people with intellectual and developmental disabilities and their families; http://www.thearc.org), or autism-specific advocacy groups such as Autism Speaks (http://www.autismspeaks.org).

Information on local health insurance programs is also provided by states through the Affordable Care Act of 2010 (PL 111-148) and the Health Care and Education Reconciliation Act of 2010 (PL 111-152) (see http://www.healthcare.gov). These sources may provide subsidies for low- to middle-income families to purchase health insurance. Even families with incomes too high to be eligible for subsidies under the Affordable Care Act may qualify for the Child Health Insurance Program (CHIP), which provides insurance benefits to children in families that could not otherwise afford health insurance. CHIP programs are administered by the states, so ways to gain access to them varies, but information on state CHIP programs can be found athttp://kff.org/medicaid/fact-sheet/where-are-states-today-medicaid-and-chip/. Medicare and Medicaid are two other federal benefit programs that may help families pay for medical care.

Medicare   In some cases, children and adults with disabilities who would not otherwise be eligible for Medicare may qualify if a third party, perhaps a custodial grandparent, pays into Medicare. This is referred to as *third party buy-in* and is similar to purchasing private health insurance.

Medicaid   Medicaid is another possible source of health insurance for low-income families. Medicaid pays for medical care for people who do not have private health insurance and do not have the income to pay for health care. It is funded by both state and federal governments, though coverage differs across states. Some states will cover services such as occupational therapy, speech-language therapy, and dental care. Medicaid also covers certain costs, such as prescriptions and medical equipment (e.g., AAC devices, wheelchairs). In some states, residential care and respite care may be covered by Medicaid. It is important to check with your local Social Security Administration (SSA) office as well advocacy groups such as Autism Speaks and Family Voices to make sure you are aware of the maximum range of benefits offered by your state. Information can also be found at http://www.medicaid.gov/index.html

Children with Special Health Care Needs Program   The Children with Special Health Care Needs (CSHCN) program is a grant administered by the Maternal and Child Health Bureau of the U.S. Department of Health and Human Services. Each state receives funds to pay for a variety of health services to infants, children, and youth under 21 years old from low-income families. The services vary from one state to another and each state sets its own financial eligibility requirements based on the family's annual income. The program promotes an integrated system of services for infants, children, and youth who have or are at risk for chronic physical, developmental, behavioral, or emotional conditions and require health and related services of a type or amount beyond what is generally needed. The program operates at both the state and local level. Most CSHCN programs also will work with families to provide information on health insurance, health care providers, and agencies. Each state has its own coordinator for this program. Your local office of The ARC, Autism Speaks, Family Voices, or the Affordable Care Act (P.L. 111-148) will be able to help you find your local program coordinator and office. The Family-to-Family Health Information Center also provides information on a state by state basis (see http://www.familyvoices.org/page?id=0034).

Supplementary Income Support The primary federal program designed to support children with disabilities from low-income households is housed in the SSA. Families of children with ASD who have low incomes may be eligible for Supplemental Security Income (SSI; http://www.ssa.gov/ssi/). These funds can be requested by completing the Child Disability Report online (http://www.ssa.gov/forms/ssa-3820.pdf) and sending any relevant medical records the family has to the local office of the SSA. The SSA then evaluates the claim, based on family income and the severity of the child's disability. If approved, the family can receive supplementary income to help cover expenses incurred for the care of the child, such as therapy not provided by the LEA, transportation to therapy, or assistive devices. The SSA also has a parent-friendly publication, *Social Security Benefits for Children* (http://www.ssa.gov/pubs/EN-05-10026.pdf), which lists resources, contact numbers, and information on government-funded programs as well as for CHIP. Table 5.1 highlights the differences between Social Security Disability Insurance (SSDI) and SSI.

Developmentally Disabled Assistance and Bill of Rights Act of 2000 The Developmentally Disabled Assistance and Bill of Rights Act of 2000 (PL 106–402) states that individuals with developmental disabilities and their families should have access to community-based services and supports to promote opportunities for independence, productivity, and inclusion. Title I of the act establishes four components: State Councils on Developmental Disabilities; Protection and Advocacy (P&A) Systems; University Centers for Excellence in Developmental Disabilities Education, Research, and Service; and Projects for National

Table 5.1. The difference between Social Security Disability Insurance (SSDI) and Supplemental Security Income (SSI)

	SSDI	SSI
Eligibility	An individual who has a disability or is blind must have paid Social Security taxes to become insured for benefits.	An adult or child who has a disability or is blind must meet all of the following categories: • Have limited income • Have limited resources • Be a U.S. citizen or national or belong in one of certain categories of aliens • Live in the United States or Northern Mariana Islands
Payment	The monthly disability benefit amount is based on the Social Security earnings record of the insured worker.	The monthly payment is based on need and varies up to the maximum federal benefit rate. Some states add money to federal SSI payments.
Medical coverage	The worker will automatically get Medicare coverage after receiving disability benefits for 2 years.	Beneficiaries in most states are automatically eligible for Medicaid.
Complete explanation of the benefit	SSDI	SSI

Source: http://ssa.gov.

Significance. The P&A system protects the legal and human rights of individuals with developmental disabilities within each state and U.S. territory and can assist families who are unable to afford the legal fees for an IDEA due process hearing. Additional information can be found at http://www.acl.gov/Programs/AIDD/DDA_BOR_ACT_2000/Index.aspx

CONCLUSION

A wide range of services are available to help families and their children with ASD. These agencies sometimes face their own challenges. Many are means-tested and have restrictions based on family income. Bureaucracies can be slow to respond to inquiries and requests, even when the issues seem urgent to you. You may encounter service providers, as you could in any professional transaction, who fail to meet your expectations. Administrators of these services are usually sympathetic to parents and work hard to achieve good outcomes for students, but they have to meet budget goals and often have fewer resources available than they would like, with a lot of people clamoring for what little is available.

Remember that your child is at his or her best when you are physically and emotionally at your best. You may feel desperate to get your young child with ASD off to the best start possible, and the most effective way to accomplish this is through a strong educational and therapeutic program. Still, being angry with the people working with your child—even if you have a right to be—won't create the most nurturing atmosphere for learning. Being agitated and upset can agitate and upset your child. Of course it is important to advocate for the finest program possible in a top facility with highly trained and talented people to work with your child. But remember that children can thrive in a surprisingly broad range of circumstances. What looks one way to you may look different to a child with ASD, who often has preferences that differ from others. The point is that your child may be able to thrive in a broader range of settings than you expect. If you aren't happy with a program, then give it a specified amount of time, keep records of the child's performance, and evaluate whether progress is being made. If it is, and your child is reasonably content, then the program may be just what he or she needs.

Try to get to know your team, talk to them about their goals and methods, and ask them about things that make you uncomfortable. You may find these interactions reassuring; team members may have reasons for doing what they do, even though it might not be what you expect. Attempt to foster positive, collaborative relationships with the professionals involved in ASD services for the sake of your own equilibrium and that of your child. Getting caught up in feelings of irritation will make you more anxious and unhappy and less able to enjoy and enrich your child's development.

The development of most children with ASD is controlled to a large extent by inborn capabilities, just like the development of other children. Yes, treatment makes a difference; and yes, better, more extensive, more consistent, more evidence-based, more focused, more thoughtful, and more expertly delivered treatment makes an even bigger difference. It's unlikely, however, that any amount or quality of treatment will change the fundamental nature of your child with ASD. Treatment can increase appropriate, useful behaviors and decrease dangerous, unconventional, or troubling behaviors. Nonetheless, treatment is not a cure, regardless of how early it starts, how long it goes on, or how good it is for your child. If your child is showing growth and improvement, even if it isn't as fast or as broad as you would like, we encourage you to work patiently and cooperatively with your team. This suggestion is not for the team's benefit but for the sake of your own state of mind and the important ways that it can affect your child.

Sample Individualized Family Service Plan (IFSP)

Early Intervention Program Individualized Family Service Plan

Child's name: Niko	Date of birth: 9/24/2009	Date of IFSP meeting: 1/25/2011	IFSP type: Initial
IFSP conducted by: Meeting with parents	IFSP effective start date: 1/26/2011	IFSP effective end date: 7/25/2011	

Child's Present Level of Functioning and How Your Child Is Doing

Physical (small muscles, big muscles, hearing, vision, and health status):

Niko is demonstrating low muscle tone, which is limiting his age-appropriate movements. He is not able to effectively move for any great distance to obtain toys or get to where he wants to be. He only supports his weight on his legs for short periods of time with assistance and is not demonstrating any independent walking. Niko also is not demonstrating good fine motor control and immature grasp patterns. An occupational therapy supplemental evaluation is recommended to further assess his fine motor skills. Supportive seating also may be beneficial. Niko exhibited a significant hearing loss based on the results of the hearing test, and his parents should consider using hearing aides for Niko.

Cognitive (thinking and reasoning skills):

Niko is experiencing difficulty with his low muscle tone and this is affecting his cognitive abilities. He is unable to obtain, hold, and activate age-appropriate toys. He is not demonstrating good visual tracking skills, and the development of simple cause-and-effect relationships is not yet present. Niko does have appropriate interactions with his parents and demonstrates the ability to participate in simple play with adult assistance. He shows happiness when playing with his mother and father and he has recently begun to wave "bye bye" but does not always make eye-contact when doing so.

From New York State Department of Health. (2014). *New York state early intervention program individualized family service plan.* Albany, NY: Author; adapted by permission of the New York State Department of Health. Retrieved from http://cma.com/wp-content/uploads/2014/08/NYEISSampleIFSP.pdf

Communication (talking and understanding language):

Niko is demonstrating a greater than 40% delay in the area of communication. He is not able to consistently follow simple one-step directions such as, "give me." He also does not demonstrate an understanding of age-appropriate language. Expressively he is only making simple utterances and only has two to three approximations of words and is unable to move his mouth in order to make all age-appropriate sounds. Niko is able to make a variety of vowel sounds and demonstrates inflection in his voice to show if he is happy, sad, mad, and so forth. His overall low muscle tone is contributing to his delays in expressive language and an evaluation by a speech-language pathologist with oral motor expertise is recommended.

Social-emotional (play skills and interacting with others):

Niko is demonstrating a greater than 40% delay in the social-emotional area. He is not able to appropriately play with toys due to low muscle tone and also is not maintaining eye contact for an appropriate amount of time. Sitting up is difficult for him and impacts his ability to play on the floor and to sit in a small chair to play with Play-Doh. Niko also is not able to move around independently or meet his own wants and needs by getting things for himself or asking for them because his language is delayed. This is contributing to his frustration level, and he will often have tantrums to try to convey what he wants. Mom is concerned because it seems like at times Niko does not hear her when she is calling to him and will often not react to something until it is directly in his line of sight.

Adaptive (self-help, feeding, dressing):

Niko has low muscle tone, which is affecting his ability to support himself in a seated position and maintain head control. He is not yet able to hold his own bottle, finger-feed himself, or begin to hold a utensil to feed himself. Niko also has difficulty maintaining his balance and is not able to effectively move around independently, which is affecting his ability to get his wants and needs met because he needs an adult to move him to be able to get to desired places and objects. Niko is demonstrating a greater than 2 standard deviation delay in the development of his adaptive and self-help skills.

Service authorization type: Assistive Technology Device

Service type: Assistive Technology Device

Intensity/method: N/A

Vendor name: Assisted Technologies Unlimited

Durable Medical Equipment description: Positioning seat for people with special orthopedic needs for use in vehicles (prior approval required for individuals younger than 2 years old or older than 10 years old) (up to 60 inches)

DME quantity: 1

Non-DME device name: N/A

Non-DME device description: N/A

Non-DME authorization amount: 0

Service authorization type: Evaluations

Service type: Nonphysician supplemental evaluation—occupational therapist

Intensity/method: Supplemental evaluation

Location: Child's home

Provider: Albany County Department of Health

Projected start date: 1/26/2011

Projected end date: N/A

Evaluation date: 3/31/2011

Evaluation domain: Physical

Service authorization type: General service authorizations

Service type: Audiology

Intensity/method: Extended home/community-based individual/collaborative visit

Frequency: 3 x IFSP period

Length (minutes/visit): 75

Location: Child's home

Provider: Albany County Department of Health

Projected start date: 1/26/2011

Projected end date: N/A

Per day limit: 1

Make-up visits for the IFSP period: 1

Covisits for the IFSP period: 3

If group visits, then enter the type of group: N/A

Service type: Family training

Intensity/method: Extended home/community-based individual/collaborative visit

Frequency: 12 x IFSP period

Length (minutes/visit): 75

Location: Child's home

Provider: Albany County Department of Health

Projected start date: 1/26/2011

Projected end date: N/A

Per day limit: 1

Make-up visits for the IFSP period: 1

Covisits for the IFSP period: 3

If group visits, then enter the type of group: N/A

Service type: Physical therapy

Intensity/method: Basic home/community-based individual/collaborative visit

Frequency: 2 x a week

Length (minutes/visit): 45

Location: Child's home

Provider: Albany County Department of Health

Projected start date: 1/26/2011

Projected end date: N/A

Per day limit: 1

Covisits for the IFSP period: 6

Service type: Special instruction

Intensity/method: Basic home/community-based individual/collaborative visit

Frequency: 1 x a week

Length (minutes/visit): 45

Location: Child's home

Provider: Albany County Department of Health

Projected start date: 1/26/2011

Projected end date: N/A

Per day limit: 1

Make-up visits for the IFSP period: 6

Covisits for the IFSP period: 6

If group visits, then enter the type of group: N/A

Service type: Speech-language

Intensity/method: Basic home/community-based individual/collaborative visit

Frequency: 2 x a week

Length (minutes/visit): 45

Location: Child's home

Provider: Albany County Department of Health

Projected start date: 1/26/2011

Projected end date: N/A

Per day limit: 1

Make-up visits for the IFSP period: 6

Covisits for the IFSP period: 6

If group visits, then enter the type of group: N/A

Service type: Applied behavior analysis

Intensity/method: Basic home/community-based individual/collaborative visit

Frequency: 4 x a week

Length (minutes/visit): 45

Location: Child's home

Provider: Albany County Department of Health

Projected start date: 1/26/2011

Projected end date: N/A

Per day limit: 1

Make-up visits for the IFSP period: 6

Covisits for the IFSP period: 6

If group visits, then enter the type of group: N/A

Assistive technology device needs

Assistive technology device (ATD) name: iPad Tap to Talk

Reason for ATD needed to attain IFSP goals: to develop two-way communication and requests

Natural environments

Are all services being provided in child's natural environment? Yes

If "no," please explain:

If any service is being provided in group setting without typically developing peers, then explain why the IFSP team agrees this is appropriate:

If the child is in child care, then list ways the qualified professionals will train child care providers to accommodate the needs of the child:

Programs or services other than early intervention

List non-early intervention services that are needed by the child and family:

May need assistance for family to learn American Sign Language and use of iPad.

Public programs child and family may be eligible for, such as Child Health Plus; Medicaid; Women, Infants, and Children; lead programs; Temporary Assistance for Needy Families; housing; waiver program (indicate if a referral will be made):

Family may need referral to appropriate waiver programs in the future.

Where does your child spend most of his or her time during a typical day (child's current setting)? Home

Did family consent to include concerns, priorities, and resources in their IFSP? Yes

Family strengths, concerns, priorities, and resources

Niko's family has a good family support network, but they have limited ability to help care for Niko or his twin sister, who has also been referred to early intervention. The family lives in a small split-level home that is very crowded and does not allow for large equipment or provide an area to facilitate a lot of movement activities. Niko's Mom and Dad have expressed that they would like assistance with finding specialty doctors that can work with Niko as needed. In addition, the family would like information on hearing loss and what they can do to become more aware of Niko's special needs. The family only has one vehicle, so transportation to appointments for Niko can be difficult.

Transportation needs

Is transportation needed? Yes

Is the child's caregiver able to provide transportation? Caregiver cannot provide

If no, please explain: Family only has one vehicle

Respite resources

Is family eligible for other sources of respite? No

If "yes," what sources:

Has family applied for this source of respite? N/A

If yes, date of application:

What is the status of this application? N/A

If family has not applied for this source of respite, please explain: N/A

Desired changes/outcomes—include methods, activities, and strategies to achieve desired outcomes (timeliness for completion, criteria and procedures to determine if progress is being made toward the achievement and whether modifications or revisions of the outcomes or services is necessary):

1. Niko will improve his head and trunk control as well as his overall strength and low tone, which will allow him to crawl on all fours and bear weight on his legs in order to get the toys he would like to play with. Activities by the early intervention team to promote this outcome will include strengthening and positioning activities such as placing Niko on all fours and encouraging him to move appropriately toward a toy he enjoys. The team will know they have been successful when Niko can successfully crawl across the living room on all fours to get a toy he wants to play with and when Niko is able to stand bearing weight on his legs next to the coffee table and play with a toy.

2. Niko will be able to pick up finger foods with an appropriate pincher grasp and correctly hold a spoon, bringing it to his mouth. Activities by the early intervention team to promote this outcome will include providing Niko with finger foods that he can practice picking up as well as providing him with opportunities to successfully feed himself with a spoon during mealtimes. The team will know they have been successful when Niko is able to feed himself Cheerios or other small finger food by picking them with an appropriate pincer grasp as well as successfully scooping applesauce or other thicker foods with a spoon and feeding himself during mealtime.

3. Niko will begin to consistently use more single words to get his wants and needs met. Activities by the early intervention team to promote this outcome will include teaching Niko to routinely use single words to ask for things he wants, rather than screaming. The team will know they have been successful when Niko uses single words on a regular basis, such as calling for "mama" or asking for "milk" and other common objects, and has decreased his tantrums and screaming.

4. Niko will be evaluated for hearing aids. Activities by the early intervention team to promote this outcome will include assisting the family as needed to gain access to an evaluation to see if hearing aids are needed to address Niko's hearing loss. The team will know they have been successful when Niko is fitted for hearing aids or the need for hearing aids has been ruled out.

5. Niko will begin to play with age-appropriate toys and play simple games. Activities by the early intervention team to promote this outcome will include providing Niko with opportunities to play with simple cause-and-effect toys and encouraging him to be able to interact with them as well as playing simple games such as Pat-a-cake and Peekaboo with Niko. The team will know they have been successful when Niko shows that he can appropriately interact with age-appropriate toys, such as pushing the buttons to make a character appear and participating in simple games with his parents.

Steps to support potential transition to the Committee on Preschools Special Education (CPSE) or other services

Date transition discussed with parents: N/A

Steps to help child adjust and function in a new setting: N/A

Did parent consent to allow qualified personnel to prepare for child's transition: N/A

If "yes," then enter procedures to allow qualified personnel to prepare for child's transition:

Did parent consent to transmit info to CPSE (including evaluation and IFSP): N/A

If "yes," then enter date transmitted:

_____ **Family agrees to incorporate the transition plan (either to CPSE or other services) in their IFSP—see separate attachment(s)**

Additional IFSP comments: Family has requested information on learning sign language

People who participated in development of this IFSP (meeting attendees):

Mom, Dad, early intervention evaluation team, and early intervention official

Other meeting participants: N/A

_____ **I give my consent to share information contained in this IFSP with all IFSP team members**

Parent/caregiver signature: _____ **Date:** _____

Parent/caregiver signature: _____ **Date:** _____

Early intervention official/designee: _____ **Date:** _____

Service coordinator: _____ **Date:** _____

Other: _____ **Date:** _____

Other: _____ **Date:** _____

Other: _____ **Date:** _____

Sample Individualized
Family Educational Plan (IEP)

STUDENT INFORMATION

NAME: Jessa

COUNTRY: United States

AGE: 4 years 8 months

SCHOOL: PS5078

PARENTS: Gary and Elizabeth

DISABILITY: Autism spectrum disorder

NATIVE LANGUAGE: English   GRADE: First

DATE OF IEP: March 30, 2015

ANNUAL REVIEW DATE: March 30, 2016

TYPE OF IEP:

☑ Initial
☐ Triennial
☐ Annual review
☐ Modified

☑ Draft until signed by parents.

For initial IEP, parent signature on the IEP indicates consent for provision of services.

Special education services (direct services to student)

Type of service	Location	Anticipated frequency	Time	Start date	End date	Service provider and/or funding source
Speech-language therapy	Pull out	2 x week	40 minutes	April 1, 2015	March 31, 2016	School speech-language pathologist (SLP)
Occupational therapy	General education classroom	2 x week	40 minutes	April 1, 2015	March 31, 2016	School occupational therapist (OT)

Consultation (indirect services to school/community personnel and parent only)

Service provider	Anticipated frequency	Time	Start date	End date	Service provided to	Funding source
Speech-language consultant	1 x every 8 weeks	60 minutes	April 1, 2015	March 31, 2016	Preschool teachers and SLP	ASD Nest Program
Behavior consultant	1 x every 8 weeks	60 minutes	April 1, 2015	March 31, 2016	Preschool teachers	
Parent workshop	2 per year	120 minutes	April 1, 2015	March 31, 2016	Preschool autism spectrum disorder (ASD) Nest parents	

Signatures:

_____   _____
Parent/guardian   Special education coordinator

Adapted from the U.S. Department of Defense Education Activity. (2005). DoDEA Form 2500.13-G-F26: Individualized education program (IEP). Alexandria, VA: Author. Retrieved from http://www.dodea .edu/Curriculum/specialEduc/upload/DoDEAForm2500-13-G-F26.pdf

Accommodations/Special Considerations

Physical education: Physical education integrated into first grade curriculum

Modifications required:

Transportation: N/A

Modifications required:

Schoolwide standardized testing:

❑ Student will participate without accommodations

❑ Student will participate with accommodations

☑ Testing not required for this grade level (kindergarten, first, second, and 12th grades)

❑ Student will participate in an alternate assessment

Accommodations:

Special factors the IEP team has determined the student requires. Each "Y" (yes) must be addressed on a goal page.

Braille	No	Limited English proficiency	No
Behavior	No	Communication needs	No
Assistive technology	No		

Consideration of extended school year

Additional data is needed in order to make this determination by: _____

☑ Documentation does not support the need for extended school year services.

Record shows student's inability to recoup skills within a reasonable time following regression and recommends extended school year services (attach documentation).

Comment:

Accommodations/modifications in general and special education

Goals and Objectives

AREA: Communication

NEED: Receptive and expressive language, feeding

PRESENT LEVEL OF PERFORMANCE: In September 2015, Jessa scored at the third percentile in auditory comprehension, the 10th percentile in expressive communication, and the fourth percentile in total language score on the Preschool Language Scale-3. She has continued to expand her vocabulary and length of utterance and is making progress on retelling a simple story. She continues to have difficulty with her phonics and making letter-sound connections. She is beginning to answer simple questions but continues to have difficulty recalling a simple sequence of events. She is narrating her play but cannot retell a simple story. Dietary intake and range of foods have increased but continue to be an area of concern.

SERVICE PROVIDER(S): SLP

ANNUAL GOAL: Jessa will develop and increase her expressive language skills.

Short-term objectives	Mastery criteria
Will tell a simple three-part story using pictures or miniatures	4 out of 5 trials
Will use adjectives when requesting	7 out of 10 trials
Will use four different adjectives when describing what she sees in a book	

ANNUAL GOAL: Jessa will develop her understanding of language for concepts and different verbs.

Short-term objectives	Mastery criteria
Will understand: long, tall, short	8 out of 10 trials
Will follow three-part directions	3 of 5 trials
Will understand the simple negative	4 of 5 trials
Will answer interrogatives with no pictures in front of her: who, what, where	80% accuracy
Will answer where, who, and what questions related to places, people, or objects that are not in her immediate environment	8 out of 10 trials

ANNUAL GOAL: Jessa will develop her social play skills.

Short-term objectives	Mastery criteria
Will carry out at least three sequences of imaginary play and will comment on her own actions	4 of 5 trials
Will take turns during free play outside	8 of 10 opportunities

Goals and Objectives

ANNUAL GOAL: Jessa will demonstrate growth in functional language.

Short-term objectives	Mastery criteria
Will express wants and needs using adjectives and with increased length of utterance	5 times daily, 5 consecutive days
Will increase length of utterances and use conjunctions to join sentences	
Will label pictures (e.g., Which one has a door? Home)	18 out of 20 trials
Will identify objects found in environment	18 out of 20 trials

ANNUAL GOAL: Jessa will improve semantic skills by strengthening classification and categorization skills.

Short-term objectives	Mastery criteria
Will classify words/concepts by category, function, and common characteristics	80% accuracy
Will increase use of prepositions: under, on, and next to	90% accuracy

ANNUAL GOAL: Jessa will improve syntax and morphology.

Short-term objectives	Mastery criteria
Will demonstrate use of nouns and regular plural nouns	80% accuracy
Will use verb forms: regular present tense, regular past	70% accuracy

ANNUAL GOAL: Jessa will increase mean length of response.

Short-term objectives	Mastery criteria
Will produce simple sentences of an MLU of five	90% accuracy
Will produce declarative sentences	80% accuracy
Will produce compound sentences	60% accuracy

ANNUAL GOAL: Jessa will improve auditory and phonological skills.

Short-term objectives	Mastery criteria
Will imitate rhythm	6 out of 8 trials
Will sit for storytime with minimal verbal prompts from the teacher	90% of the time
Will perform an action when she hears a certain sound or word	90% of the time
Will discriminate and identify at least 12 environmental sounds	80% accuracy

Goals and Objectives

AREA: Gross motor and handwriting (fine motor)

NEED: Sensory behaviors; self-help skills and fine motor for handwriting

PRESENT LEVEL OF PERFORMANCE: Jessa has adequate body awareness but exhibits sensory defensiveness. She avoids getting her face/nose wiped and becomes agitated when having her hair washed and nails trimmed. She does not like her hands to be wet or messy. She does not like to wear shoes and complains when her clothes are scratchy. She enjoys splashing during water play. She frequently bumps into objects. She walks on her toes when she isn't wearing shoes. She enjoys physical activity. She avoids eye contact with strangers but not with familiar adults and teachers. She frequently has difficulty eating in noisy environments. She resists all but a few food choices and refuses to try new foods. She has improved her pincer grip but has difficulty forming letters and tends to press lightly.

SERVICE PROVIDER(S): OT

ANNUAL GOAL: Jessa will decrease sensory defensive behaviors.

Short-term objectives	Mastery criteria
Decrease sensory defensive behaviors during real-life situations with verbal prompt	8 out of 10 times
Participate in activities requiring tactile modalities at school upon request	As needed
Independently self-modulate sensory input across two settings using visual supports	7 out of 10 times
Utilize the break area in the classroom	

ANNUAL GOAL: Jessa will develop her grooming skills.

Short-term objectives	Mastery criteria
Tolerate washing and drying of hands and face upon request	8 out of 10 times

ANNUAL GOAL: Jessa will develop her eating skills.

Short-term objectives	Mastery criteria
Tolerate various types/textures of food within range expected for developmental level	4 out of 5 times
Eat at a proper speed in a variety of settings with verbal prompt on a daily basis	9 out of 10 consecutive days

ANNUAL GOAL: Jessa will develop her handwriting.

Short-term objectives	Mastery criteria
Will use the appropriate spacing, letter formation, and different size letters (large and small)	4 out of 5 times
Will work on line accuracy and draw basic straight-line and round shapes	
Will consistently form numbers and lowercase letters	
Will correctly place numbers and lowercase letters in relation to the line	

Least Restrictive Environment

In making the program decision, the following factors were considered by the IEP team in selecting the least restrictive environment.

 __X__ Placement of the student is based on his or her individual needs.

 __X__ Student is educated with students who do not have disabilities to the maximum extent appropriate.

 __X__ Removal from general education only when the nature and severity of the student's educational needs are such that education in the general education program with supplementary support and services cannot be achieved satisfactorily.

 __X__ Participation with general education students in school activities to the maximum extent appropriate.

 __X__ Placement is as close as possible to the student's home or in the school he or she would attend if he or she did not have a disability.

Justification for placement: Explanation of the extent, if any, to which the student will not participate with peers without disabilities. Describe how the student's disability affects his or her involvement and progress in the general curriculum. For preschool children, indicate how the child's disability affects his or her participation in appropriate activities.

The social-communicative delays affect Jessa's ability to express her needs, in the school setting, at home, and on the playground.

Student progress: Parents will be informed of their child's progress in meeting the goals of his or her IEP on the same timeline as students without disabilities.

Method by which the student's progress will be reported: In accordance with private preschool practices

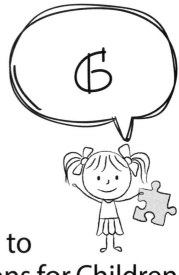

What Do Families Need to Know About Interventions for Children with Autism Spectrum Disorder

This chapter is designed to help you understand some of the issues and options for treating social-communication difficulties in your young child with ASD. Chapter 4 talked about the professionals who may be involved in this intervention. This chapter begins by outlining the when, where, what, and why of early intervention for children with ASD, and includes a consideration of the importance of scientific evidence in selecting intervention practices. Next, this chapter and the following one outline the approaches to improving social-communication that you are likely to encounter in early intervention programs for your child and talk about the broad categories used to classify interventions. This chapter also focuses on discussing how to evaluate the scientific evidence for these interventions to help you learn what questions to ask in order to determine the scientific support for treatment procedures that may be proposed for your child. But first, let's hear from Sara, Noah's mother.

My husband, Andreas's nephew, has autism, and we knew there was a possibility that Noah might receive a diagnosis of ASD. We noticed that Noah was not using sounds or gestures to communicate when he was 15 months old. He would take us by the hand and guide us to what he wanted, or he would just get the item himself. He was more interested in playing with my necklace than looking at me and generally avoided looking at people to communicate his needs. He loves the movie *Frozen* but would want to watch it all day if we let him. If we tried to get him to watch something else, then he would become very upset and cry. He doesn't like noisy places and is easily disturbed in his sleep, which is just like his Dad. We knew that early intervention was important, and we spoke to our pediatrician about our concerns. She referred us for an assessment. Noah received a diagnosis of ASD at 18 months, and we wanted to start intervention right away. Even though we were somewhat prepared for the fact that he might have autism, we were still very emotional and had trouble wading through all the different treatments available and figuring out where to begin. My husband and I went online and searched for autism treatments. There were over 13 million hits! How could we know which treatment would be right for Noah? It would help to understand how to sort out treatments that were effective from those that made empty promises.

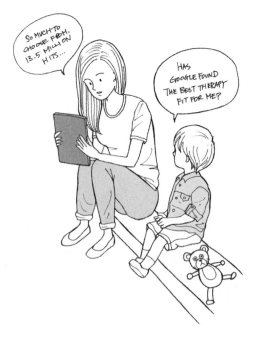

Sara's concerns may sound familiar. How can a family sift through the enormous amount of information available to find the most appropriate treatment for their child? Let's begin by addressing some basic questions.

WHEN CAN INTERVENTION BEGIN?

The simple answer is, early. The National Research Council (2001) reviewed scientific studies of autism treatments and established six common elements of best practices for intervention for children with ASD:

1. Intervention should start early in life.

2. Intervention should be intensive.

3. Intervention should include parents.

4. Intervention should be structured.

5. Interventionists should be well trained.

6. Child-to-teacher ratios should be low, and there should be a significant amount of one-to-one teaching.

These are elements to look for in any intervention program for a young child with ASD. You may be thinking, I know early intervention is important, but my child is only a baby—he's not even 2 years old. Isn't he way too young to go to school?

First, most children who receive intervention services before age 3 don't go to school in the way we usually think of it. Interventionists may come to your home to work with you and the child, or, if your child goes to child care, then services may happen there. The aim of early intervention is to see the child in the natural environment, which is where the child normally spends most of the time. If that's the home, then services will happen there.

Early interventionists understand that very young children don't learn the same way as school-age children. Early childhood specialists know that young children need a lot of sensory and motor experiences to learn and they learn best in one-to-one settings with a familiar adult.

> Early childhood specialists know that young children need a lot of sensory and motor experiences to learn and they learn best in one-to-one settings with a familiar adult.

The goals of early intervention are different from the goals of school programs. Early intervention aims to maximize the child's strengths and work on areas of need, rather than teaching the child specific knowledge. Early intervention specialists use therapeutic and educational strategies to help young children acquire daily living and adaptive skills such as feeding, toileting, moving in an age-appropriate way, and communicating. Early intervention specialists also will spend time with you as a family, teaching you how to help your child learn new skills and maintain them over time.

Early intervention is important for children with ASD because it helps them acquire skills needed to learn from teachers and peers in mainstream school settings, and it also helps to push them toward what developmental scientists call a *typical growth trajectory*. Children with ASD often have difficulty learning what other children seem to learn naturally without much obvious instruction because they tend to pay attention to things that aren't usually interesting to other children (e.g., spinning things, peering closely at small details of objects). They often pay less attention to the things that are very interesting to typically developing children, however, such as people's faces and voices and how they use objects. This pattern of intense interest in nonsocial aspects of the environment coupled with limited focus on people and what they do can lead to a slower rate of learning the social-communication skills that seem to come so effortlessly to typically developing children, such as gestures, speech, and play.

These differences may not be related to intelligence; even bright children with ASD may miss social learning opportunities due to their greater focus on nonsocial rather than social aspects of the environment. This contrasts with other kinds of developmental disabilities, such as Down syndrome. Children

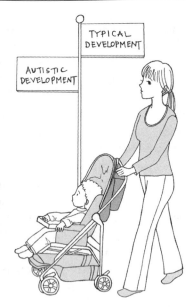

with Down syndrome may be slow in learning to talk, but when people talk to them, they are interested, pay attention, and try to interact. They get a lot of chances to hear words and see how they match up with the objects around them. They are on a typical learning trajectory but learn more slowly because of their intellectual impairment. The child with ASD, though, is less inclined to take advantage of opportunities in the environment that would support social learning, even in the presence of relatively strong cognitive capacity. Children with ASD may not look at things other people are looking at, so they won't get the chance to link words people say to the things people look at. Instead, a child with ASD may prefer to look at the wheel of a toy train or a small part of an object rather than the object as a whole. The more time spent looking at the wheel, the fewer chances there are to notice that Mom is saying, "The train says 'choo-choo'" and learn what a *train* is and its associated word. The child may be missing an opportunity to connect the word *train* to the toy Mom is pointing out. People may even begin to talk less than they would to other children because they get tired of not being listened to (behaviorists call this process *extinction*). Yet, the brain of the child with ASD is getting a lot of input about the wheel on the toy train; this child may know a lot about the differences among wheels on a lot of different toys and may even become an expert about wheels. All that brain power being used to learn about wheels is not being used to learn about people and things they find important.

In a way, the brain is like a muscle: The more it is used, the stronger it gets. Children on typical developmental trajectories find people and the things they do fascinating. Children pay a lot of attention to people and try to imitate them, which provides practice, helps them get new information about people and their actions, and strengthens the brain processes that do this type of learning about people so that these processes begin to work faster and more efficiently. Future learning that uses these processes becomes quicker and easier.

"People-learning" or *social brain processes* tend not to get as much exercise in children with ASD. The result is twofold—the child with ASD has acquired less information about people and social skills and struggles to understand other people's behavior, which can make people seem confusing and unpredictable. This kind of social discomfort makes it even *more* appealing for the child with ASD to focus attention on things that feel more familiar, which can result in spending even more time and energy learning about wheels. This

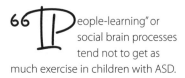

"People-learning" or social brain processes tend not to get as much exercise in children with ASD.

cycle puts the child on an atypical trajectory; the child with ASD is not just learning more slowly than other children, but is developing different, less functional skills that can cause development to veer even further off the typical path.

The opportunity to redirect your child's development toward a more typical trajectory is one reason why early intervention is so important. By providing exciting, engaging activities that focus the child's attention on people early on, there is a chance to stave off some of the effects of an atypical developmental trajectory. If children with ASD can be pushed closer to the path of typical development, then they will not only have more opportunities to learn skills but will also have more chances to exercise and strengthen the brain processes that develop social skills and understanding.

Parents of children with ASD who are 18–24 months old who worry about their children's development can seek an evaluation from a multidisciplinary team with experience diagnosing ASD sooner rather than waiting and hoping the child will grow out of the problem. An evaluation won't hurt, and every state provides publically funded developmental evaluations for children under 3 years of age. If ASD is diagnosed, then intervening early not only leaves more time to teach skills before school age but also presents the possibility providing more adaptive experiences to exercise and strengthen the brain's social learning processes.

WHERE DO SERVICES TAKE PLACE?

IDEA 2004 states that early intervention programs should take place in the child's "natural environment." For many children under 3, this will mean in the home, and therapists from birth-to-3 service agencies often will come to the home to work with children and their families. Some children attend child care due to parents' work schedules, and child care centers are natural environments for young children, too. Some birth-to-3 agencies create special education centers for children under 3 years old in which the children attend an early intervention center several days a week and receive preschool experiences with peers and trained teachers, along with individual sessions with therapists. Parents may also spend time at these facilities and be able to observe and participate in their child's program as well as receive training from staff on how to carry over activities at home. Any of these arrangements, or a combination of them, can be effective ways to provide early intervention services. Parents have the right to expect that their service providers will meet with them regularly to update them on their child's progress and will help them find ways to carry over the intervention activities in daily routines in the home or child care setting when therapists are not around.

WHAT WILL MY CHILD NEED TO LEARN?

Before we answer this question, we need to go back to our discussion about assessment. Every young child diagnosed with ASD should receive an intensive evaluation before an intervention program can be designed, which should ideally be delivered within a multidisciplinary framework involving professionals from several different disciplines. Your child's evaluation will probably consist of a diagnostic assessment to determine whether ASD is present, as well as an assessment of current strengths and needs in order to identify individual goals for the educational plan. In addition to special education services, family education, speech-language therapy, occupational therapy, and physical therapy are the kinds of services that are typically part of early intervention. All of these services will be aimed at addressing the core symptoms of ASD—the social-communication, cognitive, emotional, self-help, and motor impairments that are characteristic of this syndrome, as well as any issues that might be particular to your child.

Most children with ASD have needs across several developmental areas. The National Research Council's report on *Educating Children with Autism* (Lord & McGee, 2001) identified eight major areas of development that commonly need to be addressed in educational programs for young children with ASD:

1. Motor imitation

2. Joint attention

3. Play

4. Using gestures

5. Vocal imitation (making speech sounds)

6. Looking to learn (eye contact and gaze management)

7. Listening to learn (attention to speech)

8. Spontaneous communication

    • Using signs and pictures (AAC) to communicate

    • Using sounds, words, word approximations, phrases, and sentences to communicate

The educational plans of most children with ASD will have goals and activities in each of these critical areas.

WHY IS IT IMPORTANT TO SELECT EVIDENCE-BASED PRACTICES?

Using evidence-based practices means that intervention procedures are tested in a scientific way to determine whether they are effective. Box 6.1 defines some of the terms used to evaluate intervention procedures and decide whether they meet scientific standards of evidence.

Evidence-Based Practice Terms

Antecedent-based intervention (ABI)   Reducing interfering behaviors by identifying the events, circumstances, or instructions that precede an interfering behavior and accordingly rearranging/eliminating them to lead to the reduction of the behavior.

Cognitive behavior training/intervention (CBT)   Usually used to treat symptoms of ASD such as anxiety, depression, or obsessional behavior. CBT assumes that changing thinking leads to changing behavior. This typically is used with individuals who are verbal and high functioning and aims to help individuals change beliefs and substitute negative thoughts with positive thoughts, thus decreasing emotional distress and self-defeating behavior.

Differential reinforcement   Either providing positive/desirable consequences for behaviors to increase the likelihood of the behaviors reoccurring or removing/reducing these positive/desirable consequences to reduce the likelihood of the behavior reoccurring.

Discrete trial teaching (DTT)   An instructional procedure designed to teach appropriate behavior or identified skills. Instruction involves presenting multiple trials. The following three steps are involved in each trial: teacher's instruction, the desired/expected response from the child, and the planned consequence (reinforcement).

Extinction   Aims to eliminate a behavior by eliminating the reinforcement for that behavior.

Functional behavioral assessment (FBA)   Collection of data over a given period of time by systematically observing/describing the interfering behavior and identifying the setting in which it occurs, the antecedent prior to the behavior occurring, and the consequences that follow the behavior. A hypothesis is developed from the collected data as to why the interfering behavior occurs, and a behavior intervention plan is developed and the hypothesis is tested.

Functional communication training (FCT)   Replacing interfering behaviors with a more positive functional means of communicating needs that serves the same function (e.g., using the sign for EAT rather than screaming to request for food).

Hanen's More Than Words   An in-home, individualized program to train parents to use strategies that focus on everyday activities to improve communication, to provide more mature and conventional communication, and to improve skills in understanding language and social interactions in preschool children with ASD.

Joint attention/mediated learning (JAML)   A direct, therapist-delivered intervention focused on teaching receptive and expressive joint attention behaviors by using naturalistic behavioral techniques.

(continued)

BOX 6.1 (continued)

Joint attention and symbolic play engagement regulation (JASPER)
A direct, therapist-delivered intervention focused on teaching receptive and
expressive joint attention behaviors as well as symbolic uses of objects by
using naturalistic behavioral techniques.

Milieu communication training (MCT)   Involves arranging stimuli in the
environment to create a setting that encourages children with ASD to initiate communication behavior. Targeted language behaviors can be elicited
with adult modeling and functional consequences associated with child
requests.

Modeling   The teacher/instructor demonstrates the desired behavior that
leads to imitation of the behavior by the child with ASD, which leads to
the acquisition of the imitated behavior. Modeling often is combined with
prompting and reinforcement in ABI.

Naturalistic intervention   Providing intervention and teaching skills during typical everyday settings, activities, and routines in which the learner
participates. For example, the child with ASD may learn to name body
parts or imitate the action "arms up" during bath time. Natural consequences are arranged for the targeted skills (e.g., child is tickled when
arms are raised).

Parent-implemented intervention   A technique or program is taught to parents by a therapist, who coaches the parent in implementing the intervention. The parent then carries over the techniques and strategies in the home
setting.

Peer-mediated instruction and intervention (PMII)   Social learning opportunities are set up between children with ASD and their typically developing peers to help children with ASD acquire new behavior and social-
communication skills. A teacher is present to facilitate the interaction and
teach strategies to support the engagement.

Picture Exchange Communication System (PECS)   PECS aims to teach functional communication skills with a focus on spontaneous communication.
Children are taught, through modeling, to exchange a picture for a desired
object. Subsequent teaching aims to reduce reliance on the model and
increase the complexity of the child's communication.

Pivotal Response Training (PRT)   Teaches skills that support the acquisition
of a wide range of other skills, include initiating, responding to multiple
cues, and providing motivation through a series of guided intervention
practices. Learning takes place in a variety of settings that build on the
young child's interests and initiative.

Prompting   Assistance provided by the instructor so the child is successful
and is able to engage in or acquire the target skill. Prompts can be physical, gestural, or verbal and used in combination (e.g., a verbal and physical
prompt can be combined to teach a child to sign for and say EAT).

Reinforcement   An object, activity, or circumstance that occurs after a child
engages in a desired behavior or skill that leads to the increase of the behavior over time. Or, anything you say, do, or provide after a child exhibits
a behavior that increases the likelihood that the behavior will continue to
occur in the future and even increase with time.

BOX 6.1 *(continued)*

Response interruption/redirection   This is used to reduce interfering behaviors such as odd, stereotypical motor and vocal patterns and echolalia. It involves interruption and redirection: redirecting the child's attention by saying something not related to the situation, prompting the child, or using other distracters when an interfering behavior is occurring that are designed to divert the child's attention away from the interfering behavior and result in its reduction. For example, if a child has echolalia or giggles when he or she sees a peer, then he or she can be taught instead to say "hello."

Responsive education and prelinguistic milieu teaching (RPMT)   A version of MCT developed for children who have not yet acquired verbal language. It teaches parents to respond to a child's nonverbal attempts at communication and uses therapist-delivered intervention to increase the frequency of intentional communication acts, first with gaze, gestures, and nonspeech vocalizations and later with words.

Scripting   This technique takes advantage of the tendency of children with ASD to echo what others say. It teaches the child functional recorded or written scripts for social activities, such as greeting or asking questions, then gradually fades parts of the script until the child can independently express the scripted language in appropriate situations.

Self-management   Self-management plans are used to teach students to independently complete tasks and monitor and reinforce their own behavior. Essential elements of self-management include setting goals, monitoring behavior, and evaluating progress. Students may observe their own behavior, record its occurrence on a data sheet, and evaluate progress. Students take an active role in self-reinforcement by deciding how to evaluate progress and when to deliver a reinforcer to him- or herself. This is primarily used with students with ASD who are verbal and high functioning.

Social narrative   A social narrative uses text and images to describe a social situation in detail by highlighting what will happen, the social context, and the hidden social cues and offering examples of appropriate responses for the given situation. Social narratives are individualized and can be used with adults or children with ASD.

Social skills training   This training attempts to provide children with ASD with the tools they need to successfully engage in social interactions in order to broaden their opportunities to make friends, enjoy social contact, and use social situations to enhance their overall adaptive outcome. It usually takes place in small-group settings. Its content needs to be carefully crafted to match the child's developmental level. Social skills training for young children might focus on simple acts such as greetings, joining a peer in play with a toy, or sharing. Teaching methods might include practicing scripts for greeting or using video modeling to observe how typically developing peers greet each other, then practicing the same strategies.

Speech-generating device (SGD)/voice output communication aid (VOCA)   These are augmentative and alternative communication devices that speak electronically when a picture is selected or when text is typed into a software program.

(continued)

BOX 6.1 (continued)

Structured playgroups   These are a form of peer-mediated intervention in which children with ASD are encouraged to participate in play with typically developing peers while being coached by a therapist. The adult provides materials, starts play, or joins in with children's play to offer some direction or guidelines. Structured play activities usually have a clear endpoint, such as putting together a puzzle. They may involve a well-known script to enact, such as going to fast-food restaurant, and may use a visual schedule to support the sequence of activities.

Structured work systems   These are a technique drawn from the Treatment and Education of Autistic and related Communication Handicapped Children (TEACCH) comprehensive program. They are similar to structured play in that the child is given a clear sequence of activities to follow, with coaching from an adult and/or a visual schedule. The activities, however, include some functional, goal-oriented job, such as putting away groceries.

Task analysis   Breaking down an activity or behavior into small, manageable steps in order to either assess what the learner can do or to teach the necessary skills. For example, washing hands can be broken down into six or more steps.

Time delay   Providing the learner with extra time or a brief delay after he or she is asked to engage in behavior or demonstrate a skill prior to providing additional instructions or prompts. The goal is to support the learner in becoming more independent and less reliant on the prompts. This technique is often used in milieu teaching approaches.

Video modeling   The child is shown a video of the expected behavior or skill to assist in learning it. The video is either of the child caught using the skill or of a peer demonstrating the skill.

Visual support   Any visual display that can include written words, pictures, symbols, or concrete items to support the learner in acquiring skills, understanding the routine/schedule, and helping to increase appropriate behaviors and/or reduce challenging behaviors. Examples of visual supports include visual schedules, pictures of task analysis for daily living, labels in the environment, and organizational systems.

There are several comprehensive curricula for young children with ASD that are designed to address all of the aspects of development identified by the National Research Council and have been the subject of some scientific study (see Table 6.1). Many of these comprehensive programs, unfortunately, are offered only in specific geographic locations, so they may not be readily accessible to every child (see Figure 6.1). Even if a well-researched, comprehensive program is not available in your area, it is still possible to construct a program that addresses the major areas of development previously outlined and uses (and can show you the scientific basis of) evidence-based methods. Although it is important that the program identifies your child's individual strengths and needs, it is also wise to remember that the areas identified by the National Research Council provide a good idea of the curriculum that should guide intervention at early

Table 6.1. Comprehensive programs for treating young children with ASD with reported outcome data

Program	Age group	Web site/contact	Level of evidence*	Citation
Denver Model	3–5 years	none	II	Rogers et al. (2006)
Early Start Denver Model	9–36 months	http://www.autism speaks.org/what -autism/ treatment/ early-start -denver -model-esdm	I	Rogers and Dawson (2010)
Developmental, Individual Differences, Relationship-Based Model (DIR/Floortime)	2–6 years	http://www.icdl.com/ DIR	III	Solomon, Necheles, Ferch, and Bruckman (2007)
Douglass Developmental Disabilities Center	3–5 years	http://dddc.rutgers .edu	II	Harris and Handleman (2000)
Princeton Child Development Institute	Infant to adult	http://www.pcdi.org	II	Fenske, Zalenski, Krantz, and McClannahan (1985)
Learning Experience: An Alternative Program (LEAP)	3–6 years	http://challenging behavior.fmhi.usf .edu/explore/ webinars/6.27 .2012_tacsei_ presentation.htm	III	Hoyson, Jamieson, and Strain (1984)
Lovaas Institute	2–8 years	http://eric.ed.gov/ ?id=ED473063	II	Cohen, Amerine-Dickens, and Smith (2006)
May Institute	Infant to adult	http://www.may institute.org	III	Campbell et al. (1998)
Pivotal Response Treatment (PRT)	3–21 years	http://www.autism prthelp.com	II	Koegel and Koegel (2006)
Relationship Development Intervention (RDI)	Infant to adult	http://www.rdi connect.com	III	Gutstein, Burgess, and Montfort (2007)
Responsive Teaching	1–5 years	http://www .responsive teaching.org	III	Mahony and Perales (2005)
Social Communication, Emotional Regulation, Transactional Support (SCERTS®)	Birth to 10 years	http://www.scerts .com	III	Prizant et al. (2006)
Strategies for Teaching Based on Autism Research (STAR)	3–21 years	http://starautism support.com	III	Arick et al. (2003)
Treatment and Education of Autistic and related Communication Handicapped Children (TEACCH)	2 years to adolescence	http://teacch.com/ about-us/what-is -teacch	II	Ozonoff and Cathcart (1998)

Sources: Odom, Boyd, Hall, and Hume (2010a); Odom, Collet-Klinterberg, Rogers, and Hatton (2010b); Wagner, Wallace, and Rogers (2014).

*As outlined in Table 6.3,

    I: Well-conducted randomized controlled trial

    II: Quasi-experimental or multiple-baseline study

    III: Observational study

childhood developmental level. Most children in their early years will benefit from a program that places emphasis on these eight areas.

In addition to these comprehensive programs, a lot of research since 2000 has focused on demonstrating the efficacy of a range of less comprehensive, more targeted intervention procedures for teaching specific skills to children with ASD. A task force of researchers and clinicians wrote the National Autism Standards Report (NSR) in 2015, a comprehensive picture of the state of scientific evidence on intervention procedures that had been published in the field at that time. The task force created three categories to classify the available treatments:

1. *Established treatments:* known to be effective for individuals with autism

2. *Emerging treatments:* known to demonstrate some evidence of effectiveness as a result of single case studies, small sample studies, or quasi-experimental studies

3. *Unestablished treatments:* no published evidence of effectiveness.

Table 6.2 presents a list of practices identified by the most recent reports available as of this writing as having some degree of evidence—either established or emerging—for improving symptoms in children with ASD. These practices treat just one aspect of behavior and are usually incorporated into a more eclectic intervention program than would be found in one of the comprehensive curricula.

Although an evidence-based comprehensive curriculum can be beneficial, a program that provides a range of evidence-based specific treatment practices like those in Table 6.2 also can be effective. Before we review the practices themselves, though, we feel it is necessary to convince you how important it is when selecting an intervention to ensure there is some systematic research to back its effectiveness. Many people have ideas about what to do about ASD because the subject has been in the news a lot; some approaches are valid from a scientific standpoint and others, not so much. To make sure your child experiences an

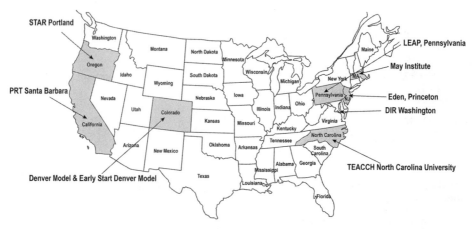

Figure 6.1. Locations for interventions for autism spectrum disorder.

Table 6.2. List of evidence-based practices

Practice*	Evidence level
Antecedent-based intervention (ABI)	Established
Cognitive behavior training/intervention (CBT)	Established
Differential reinforcement of other behaviors	Established
Discrete trial training/teaching/intervention (DTT/DTI)	Established
Extinction	Emerging
Functional behavioral assessment (FBA)	Established
Functional communication training (FCT)	Established
Hanen's More Than Words	Emerging
Joint attention/mediated learning (JAML)	Established
Joint attention and symbolic play engagement regulation (JASPER)	Established
Milieu communication training	Emerging
Modeling	Established
Naturalistic intervention	Established
Parent-implemented intervention	Emerging
Peer-mediated instruction and intervention	Emerging
Picture Exchange Communication System (PECS)	Established
Pivotal Response Training (PRT)	Established
PROMPT	Emerging
Prompting	Established
Reinforcement	Established
Response interruption/redirection	Established
Responsive education and prelinguistic milieu teaching (RPMT)	Emerging
Scripting	Emerging
Self-management	Established
Social narrative	Emerging
Social skills training	Emerging
Speech-generating device (SGD)/voice output communication aid (VOCA)	Emerging
Structured playgroups	Emerging
Structured work systems	Established
Task analysis	Established
Technology-aided instruction (e.g., iPad)	Emerging
Time delay	Emerging
Video modeling	Established
Visual support	Established

*See Box 6.1 for definitions.

Sources: Hume and Odom (2011); Wagner, Wallace, and Rogers (2014); Wong, Odom, Hume, Cox, Fettig, Kurchararczyk, Brock, Plavnick, Fleury, and Schultz (2015).

effective program, you will want to ensure that the methods used have some scientific foundation. Table 6.3 provides guidelines for the ranking quality of scientific evidence. In the section below, we'll discuss this process further.

First, although many well-intentioned people and programs aim to improve function in ASD, it takes more than good intentions to be effective. Just because a person or program is sincere and means well does not necessarily mean what they offer will help your child. Doctors in the 18th and 19th centuries who bled patients with leeches did it because they sincerely believed in the method and wanted to provide relief to their patients, but that would not be done today because science has provided us with procedures with documented effectiveness.

Make sure that the methods used in a program have some scientific foundation so that your child is exposed to the most effective program for him or her.

Second, things change over time. As your child grows, some symptoms will get better on their own, other symptoms will periodically wax and wane. These changes can happen without any intervention at all; they are part of the normal course of development. How will you know whether the changes you see are the result of your child's intervention or natural fluctuation? It can be hard without objective, systematic measurement of change that controls for some of this natural variation. When interventions are scientifically subjected to objective assessment and are shown to result in change over and above what would naturally happen, you can be confident that the intervention will do the same for your child.

Third, appearances can be deceiving because people tend to see what they expect to see. People also tend to think that a problem will get better if they focus all of their effort and attention on it. When your child starts intervention or moves to a new intervention program, it is natural to feel good about the new approach and believe it is causing improvement. Everyone is subject to this cognitive bias. This is why doctors try to have outcomes assessed by blind raters—people who don't know whether the patient got the medicine—when they study the effects of medicine. Some studies have gone so far as to give fake surgery to people to evaluate whether a particular surgical technique helps a condition, because clinicians, patients, and the patients' families naturally assume a treatment will help and they begin to see signs that it is helping. They aren't lying; it's just the natural tendency to see what is expected. Researchers try to overcome this tendency with *blinding*, or having people rate outcomes who do not know—are blind to—what intervention was used to achieve the outcome.

Carefully posing questions is another way to avoid the bias of seeing what is expected. Scientific study of intervention aims to learn not only whether a treatment causes a difference in behavior, but also whether a treatment causes more change than a comparison treatment or no treatment at all. If it doesn't cause more change than something else or nothing, then it might not be the treatment that is causing a change. It might be the fact that the child is busy for more hours

Table 6.3. Ranking quality of scientific evidence

Rank	Type(s) of studies	Characteristics
Strongest	Systematic meta-analysis	Information is pooled across several well-designed randomized controlled studies.
Strong	A well-conducted single randomized controlled trial (RCT)	• Two treatments are compared • Diagnostic instruments are valid • Participant characteristics are clearly explained • Each treatment is well-defined and addresses specific symptoms • Children are randomly assigned to groups at the start of the study • There are enough participants to find differences between treatments, if they exist • Groups are equivalent at the start • Each intervention is monitored to be sure it is delivered as intended • Measures used to assess outcome are valid and reliable • Raters are blind
Strong	Systematic review	Information from several studies that do NOT meet all the standards is pooled.
Emerging	Quasi-experimental OR multiple baseline study	Some of the criteria are met, others are not; OR only one or a few children are studied, but multiple goals (target, generalization, control) are tracked.
Emerging	Observational studies with controls	Children are not randomly assigned to groups but groups are compared.
Weak	Observational studies without controls	Only one treatment is studied; no comparison treatment.
Weakest	Expert opinions without scientific evidence	Advice is based on an expert's experience without any systematic study.

Sources: Paul and Norbury (2012); Fey and Justice (2014); Robey (2004); Wagner, Wallace, and Rogers (2013).

of the day and less able to get into difficulty, that the child likes the games a particular therapist plays and shows less atypical behavior when having fun, or that some growth that is unrelated to therapy is going on. It could also be because people around the child perceive a change due to their expectations. Doctors call these reasons the *placebo effect.* You've probably heard about it in relation to drugs, but it happens in behavior therapies, too, where it is sometimes called a *halo effect.*

For example, weighted vests often have been used as a treatment in ASD. They have been purported to provide some sort of calming effect, perhaps the way swaddling calms an infant, which increases attention and engagement and reduces maladaptive behaviors. Several systematic studies, however, have shown no effect of wearing a vest (weighted or otherwise) on time children with ASD spend in on-task, in-seat, or stereotyped behavior, or in their rousal, attention, or hyperactivity. Still, in spite of the negative results found by blind raters systematically measuring specific behaviors, parents and teachers in these studies often reported believing that the vests were helpful. These parents and teachers were not being dishonest or gullible; they were simply demonstrating the power of the halo effect. You might be thinking that wearing a weighted vest doesn't do any harm. Why not use it even if it only has a very small effect or only works on a small number of people? If there is any chance at all that it helps, then why not use a simple intervention like this one? You are probably right that it doesn't do any harm (unless your child doesn't like it for some reason and spends a lot of time and energy trying to get out of it). Even if your child accepts the vest, though, how does wearing it affect the way others react? In an inclusive class, do the other students think it is odd to wear a vest? Will they spend less time with a child who dresses oddly than they otherwise might? Do teachers believe that just wearing the vest is helping and therefore feel less compelled to make time for providing individualized instruction? Do parents believe that the vest serves as an occupational therapy program, leading them to refrain from requesting occupational therapy help with functional skills such as dressing or writing? All these subtle responses to the vest can have negative consequences and reduce the child's opportunities for social interaction and learning.

These are some of the reasons it is so crucial to use scientific evidence as a basis for selecting treatments. It's not the only basis, of course. You and your child's preferences and your team's training and access to in-service education and consultation services also will play a role. But we believe that scientific evidence should always be one element in the process of deciding how to address the needs of children with ASD. So how can the evidence needed to make these decisions be found and used?

HOW MUCH OF THE RESEARCH DO PARENTS NEED TO KNOW TO MAKE AN INFORMED DECISION ABOUT TREATMENT?

No one expects you to spend your time reading research papers, but you do need to know if there is any research that supports claims of effectiveness of an intervention you are considering. There are several criteria you can discuss with your team about the intervention methods they propose.

Peer Review

Reliable intervention practices for which there is scientifically based research are published in peer-reviewed sources. This is important to know because simply being published somewhere does not necessary mean information is scientifically valid. Peer review sets a stricter standard for information about interventions and is more likely to ensure their validity. Peer review involves having several scientists with expertise and experience on a topic—but no involvement with the study in question—independently examine a study's methods, procedures, results, and conclusions to decide if they make sense. The peer-review process usually takes 6–12 months as the reviewers make comments and suggest changes in successive drafts of an article, authors make changes, reviewers look again, and so forth, often through several rounds of review. Reviewers may ask authors to add more participants to a study, change procedures, do additional testing, modify the way results are analyzed, or rethink their conclusions. Although peer review is not perfect and reviewers can be subject to the same personal and political biases as any other human being, the process generally tends to result in higher quality research than what can be found on the Internet or in how-to books that are not subject to rigorous oversight.

"Does this intervention have any support in the peer-reviewed scientific literature?" is one question any parent can ask when presented with an intervention program for their child. If there isn't any peer-reviewed information, if all the publications about a method are written by the person who created the method, if it is published in sources without peer review, and if it provides only explanation and instructions on the method and not scientific support, then parents have a right to ask why this method is being used rather than a method that does have some basis in scientifically valid evidence. There are also some other criteria beyond the basic requirement of peer review that are helpful in establishing the quality of published evidence.

> 66 "Does this intervention have any support in the peer-reviewed scientific literature?" is one question any parent can ask when presented with an intervention program for their child.

Combining Information from Several Different Studies

Doing high-quality research on behavioral treatments is difficult and expensive. There often are small numbers of participants in the study because children who are similar to each other and match all the necessary qualifications to be in the study are hard to find; children also get sick, families may drop out along the way, and teachers leave their positions. It may be hard to get all the teachers to teach the treatments in the same, prescribed way or give all the assessments in the prescribed fashion. All of these factors contribute to the limited amount of information that's available on the effectiveness of behavioral treatments. That's why scientists sometimes try to improve the situation by combining the published information from several small studies together to see whether pooling the data that was reported will give stronger support for an intervention. This kind of study that takes the results of several smaller studies and puts them together mathematically is called a *meta-analysis* or a *systematic review*.

This method is considered strong evidence because it can reduce confusion among findings from multiple studies that focus on the same treatment and provide a bottom line interpretation that takes advantage of the strength of larger numbers than were present in any single study. To do this kind of analysis, though, there have to be quite a few individual studies published on an intervention that use similar methods and participants and also meet relatively high standards of scientific design in themselves. This situation doesn't always occur for each treatment. When it does, though, meta-analysis is a useful way to understand how well a treatment works. A study needs to show most of the following characteristics of high scientific quality in order to be a candidate for inclusion in a meta-analysis.

Comparisons   High-quality research usually systematically compares a treatment with another treatment or with periods of time spent without treatment. This is one way scientists try to solve the problem of figuring out whether change can be attributed to a treatment or just the passage of time. It is not the best practice to compare children who receive intervention with those who don't, for the reasons previously discussed; studies that do this can confuse the effects of treatment with the effects of people's expectations, particularly if the people evaluating the treatment are not blind to who was treated and who wasn't. Two kinds of high-quality comparisons are usually done for behavioral treatments.

Experimental or Quasi-Experimental Studies   Two or more treatments are contrasted, and one is often an established treatment and the other is the experimental treatment, which the authors are trying to show to be equal to or more effective than the established method. Randomized controlled trials (RCTs) are considered the highest level of this type of trial. RCTs involve comparing two treatments and randomly assigning children to treatments. Randomization is considered important because it means that the participants have an equal chance of getting assigned to either treatment, so there is little chance that something about the children in the group determines whether the treatment appears effective. Let's take an example to understand why this matters.

Suppose treatments A and B are being compared. Treatment A is offered in a clinic on the east side of town; Treatment B is offered on the west side. If children are assigned to a treatment because it is nearer to their home, then the socioeconomic characteristics of the neighborhoods might have more to do with how much children learn than the treatment does. Maybe the east side of town is wealthier, parents have more time to spend with their children, are able to talk with teachers and understand how to carry over treatment activities at home, and can provide additional tutoring outside the experimental treatment. Perhaps the west side of town is poorer and houses more recent immigrants who have limited command of English, work several jobs, have less time to spend with their children, and experience more difficulty communicating with their teachers. Children from the east side are likely to do better no matter what treatment they get; if they appear to show more growth than the contrast group on the west side, then it may not be the specific treatment that is making the difference. If children are randomly assigned to the east side or west side clinics (and provided with transportation, of course), then each child has an equal chance of getting Treatment A or B, and any difference between the treatment groups after the study will likely be the result of the treatment itself.

Making sure children in the two groups are on par at the beginning, or baseline, of the study is another element of controlled trials. Children on the east side may start out at a higher level than those on the west. It may be that they have a history of better nutrition, have had fewer and shorter episodes of ear infections that could affect their language learning because their parents could afford to take them to the doctor every time they got sick, or spent more time in intervention because their parents have better transportation and are able to get them to school more consistently. If they start off at a higher level, then they are going to end up at a higher level, regardless of what intervention they were assigned. It is very important to make sure that when children are randomized to interventions that the groups are at about the same level, on average, at the beginning of the study so it will be possible to tell at the end whether the groups show similar amounts of growth. This initial equivalence is usually established by assessing the children's baseline performance on a series of standard measures that the researchers believe are related to the outcome. For example, they will probably want to make sure both groups have about the same level of intelligence, communication, and severity of symptoms. The researchers will measure these abilities before the intervention starts and make sure the groups are well matched on each of these important baseline measures. Researchers will measure these elements again after the treatment programs are completed and determine whether the two groups showed the same or different amounts of progress relative to the baseline levels of performance.

Using blind raters is a third aspect of a controlled trial. Raters can be influenced by their unwitting cognitive biases. High-quality research will make sure that the people doing the assessments after a comparison study don't know who got which treatment so the unconscious biases can't affect their observations. Again, this is not a matter of protecting against dishonesty; it is designed to minimize the effects of the inherent tendencies to see what we expect to see. The study is referred to as *blind* when the assessors are kept unaware of the participants' treatment assignment.

Double-blind protocols often are used in medical studies in which neither the doctor nor the patient knows whether the treatment was being tested or a sugar pill was given. Double-blind studies are tough to achieve in behavioral research because the clinician who provides the intervention and the child and the family participating in intervention are likely to have some knowledge of what treatment was received. This is less of a problem if clinical assessments are administered by someone other than the therapist at baseline and outcome. Parent report measures are often also part of the pre- and posttreatment assessment, which means these measures are not blindly conducted. Remember the weighted vest experiments? Even though the blind raters found no differences between use and nonuse of vests, parents and teachers thought the weighted vests worked. This is a good example of how nonblind ratings can be problematic and make treatment research harder to interpret. Blind ratings generally are more reliable than nonblind ones, and studies that employ some or mostly blind ratings are considered of higher quality than those that do not.

Suppose your treatment team answers your first question by informing you that there are peer-reviewed studies of the treatment they are proposing. You might then want to get a sense of how high quality, and therefore how reliable, the studies are by asking the following:

- Were two treatments contrasted in the study?

- Did participants have an even chance of getting either treatment due to random assignment?

- Were the groups determined to be at the same level before treatment started?

- Were raters who assessed children after treatment blind to what treatment participants received?

- Were parent ratings used, and, if so, were parents blind to the treatment their child received?

If the studies done on the proposed treatment weren't perfect, then it doesn't mean your child shouldn't get that treatment; it is important to ask whether there might be other treatments with stronger evidence and whether these might be appropriate for your child. Remember that scientific evidence isn't the only criterion for choosing a treatment. It should be one criterion, however, and you have the right to know how good the evidence is for your team's treatment option and why they believe this treatment is the best approach for your child at this time. Then again, perhaps there are no comparison studies of the team's choice of intervention. A second level of evidence might be available.

Single-Subject Multiple-Baseline Designs   Many treatment studies do not involve the high-quality group comparisons that have been discussed. Many studies examine the response of a single individual, or a few individuals, to an intervention, particularly in the literature of ABA. Although these designs are not as strong as the group comparisons outlined in this chapter, they are legitimate forms of scientific evidence, particularly if they use the *multiple-baseline* format.

Multiple-baseline designs provide an opportunity to show that the behaviors targeted in intervention improved more than other behaviors that were not targeted during intervention. Figure 6.2 outlines the procedures for conducting a multiple-baseline single-subject research design. Identifying several intervention objectives is the first step in implementing a multiple-baseline design. The multiple-baseline procedure identifies certain objectives as targets of the intervention program. A few other behaviors are identified that the child needs to learn but are not given any intervention. These other goals are considered *control goals*.

Control goals are different enough from the targeted goals so that responses are unlikely to spread from the target goal. Goals that are similar in form to the target goals can be chosen as generalization goals and would be tracked along with the target and control goals to determine whether training is carrying over, as expected, to these similar behaviors. For example, if saying "I want . . ." were the target, then the team would probably not choose "I need . . ." as the control goal because it is quite likely that some learning from "I want..." would generalize to "I need..." Instead, they might designate "I need..." as a generalization goal, then choose "Hi, [friend's name]" as a control goal.

Gathering baseline data on the target, generalization, and control goals is the second step in the multiple-baseline procedure. Baseline measures—counting how often the child uses the targets before any instruction is given—may be taken two to three different times during the course of a few days, and the percentage of usage of the targets is averaged to determine the baseline level of performance. This level would be quite low (used less than 50% of the time) because otherwise it would not be necessary to teach the target behavior.

Providing intervention for the target, but not the control or generalization goals, is the next step. Intervention is continued until a termination criterion, such as correct usage in 80% of the opportunities offered for using the target, is met. The child's use of the target, generalization, and control goals is then assessed as it was at baseline. If use of the target and generalization goals show a significant increase over the baseline, and use of the control goal remains unchanged, then it is reasonable to conclude that the intervention made the difference in the child's use of the target form. A graph of the results could resemble Figure 6.2.

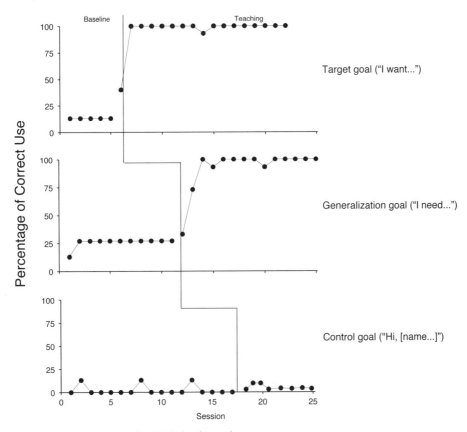

Figure 6.2.   Example outcomes of a multiple-baseline study.

If there are no controlled group comparison studies of the intervention your team is considering, then you might ask if there are any single-subject studies that have been published using the multiple-baseline method. If so, then you can ask

- Was a multiple-baseline design used?

- Were there control goals that were base-lined, left untreated, and then measured and compared with progress on the target?

- Was progress on the target and generaliza-tion goals greater than it was on the con-trol goal?

- Has there been more than one study that uses a multiple-baseline design?

> If there are no controlled group comparison studies of the intervention your team is considering, then you might ask if there are any single-subject studies that have been published using the multiple-baseline method.

If your team can answer "yes" to most of these questions, then you can con-clude that the method has emerging evidence to support it and a good chance of helping your child. If not, then ask your team why they want to use this approach in the absence of any scientific evidence and what other considerations they are using in recommending it for your child. Your aim in this process is to be a criti-cal consumer and to know what questions are reasonable to ask in order to have an informed discussion about the best approaches for your child.

You also may be concerned about methods your team is not proposing. You may have heard about a program or method from other parents or the Internet and wonder why your child isn't getting that treatment. The lack of scientific evidence behind the program may be one reason your team is not offering the treatment, despite some enthusiasm about it on the Internet. There are a lot of reasons why people may believe a treatment works when more systematic study shows it has limited value.

In addition to a lack of studies in peer-reviewed journals, other warning signs that a treatment might not be scientifically based include promises of a quick fix or total cure and a claim to treat autism itself, rather than specific symptoms. Other warning signs include a requirement to use only the treatment in question and not any oth-ers, to use only therapists who have undergone training by the originators of the methods, or to pay large sums of money for the training or the treatment itself. There are no treatments with established effectiveness known at the time of this writing that cure autism, that can't be combined with other treatments, or that can be effectively used only by a select group of individuals who charge high fees. If your team

> In addition to a lack of studies in peer-reviewed journals, other warning signs that a treatment might not be scientifically based include promises of a quick fix or total cure and a lack of treatment-specific symptoms (e.g., communication, maladaptive behavior) with the claim to treat autism itself.

is not suggesting treatments like these, then they probably have a good reason, but it never hurts to ask them to explain their reasoning. Box 6.2 offers some guidance for deciding what treatments may be appropriate for your child.

What You Need to Know to Judge the Appropriateness of a Treatment or Intervention

Seven questions to ask when evaluating an intervention approach:

1. What symptoms does the intervention address?
2. Are these symptoms high-priority targets for your child?
3. What research evidence supports this approach?
4. What are the expected outcomes?
5. How is progress systematically monitored?
6. What are the advantages and disadvantages for using this approach?
7. What are the risks involved?

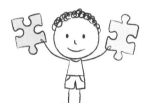

CONCLUSION

If you aren't a scientist yourself, then you may feel that this chapter has discussed more than you ever wanted to know about the conduct of behavioral research. The chapter's aim is only to help you be the most informed consumer you can be when it comes to understanding and contributing to your child's educational program. Knowing what it takes to establish a solid scientific basis for the treatments used to address symptoms of ASD will allow you to feel confident when discussing the pros and cons of various approaches with your team, to have questions ready to address some of your concerns, and to understand the answers. This knowledge should help you feel less overwhelmed by the large amount of information (and misinformation) that is so accessible in this high-tech age and more empowered to make thoughtful decisions in collaboration with the people who work with your child.

What Are the Most Effective Communication Interventions for Young Children with Autism Spectrum Disorder?

Scientific evidence is important, but it is not the only consideration when evaluating intervention programs for your child. Chapter 6 presented ideas about how you can evaluate treatments used with young children with ASD. You now know some questions you can ask when discussing programs with your intervention team. This chapter looks in more detail at some of the treatments currently available, primarily focusing on those that address the core symptom of social-communication.

Since the mid-1980s, a great deal of information has been gathered about how children with ASD learn best. One thing researchers found is that they learn somewhat differently from other children. For example, studies of young children whose language delays are not associated with ASD suggest that they usually learn effectively from interventions embedded in play and natural interactions, with clear models of language forms provided by adults and opportunities presented—without too much pressure—for children to use the models in their own speech (e.g., Hancock & Kaiser, 2006; Munro, Lee, & Baker, 2008; Warren et

Studies of young children whose language delays are not associated with ASD suggest that they usually learn effectively from interventions embedded in play and natural interactions, with clear models of language forms provided by adults and opportunities presented—without too much pressure—for children to use the models in their own speech.

al., 2006). Young children with ASD often have a different learning style, particularly in social-communication areas. They are less able to learn from natural interactions than other children because they have problems paying attention to what other people are attending to (i.e., joint attention), and they often need some additional structure to help them focus their attention on what is relevant for learning.

This chapter looks at three categories of methods that interventionists have devised to attempt to provide enhanced learning conditions for children with ASD—*ABA, developmental/pragmatic approaches,* and *relationship-based methods.* Each of these approaches is based on particular assumptions about how children learn, which we'll outline for you. Comprehensive programs within each of the three methods will be discussed, and intervention techniques that are more targeted on specific symptoms and may be used by a single therapist as one segment of a child's overall program will also be presented. Our focus will be the interventions with some degree of scientific evidence, but we'll also comment briefly on certain approaches that, in spite of having little or no scientific basis, are still commonly employed.

PRINCIPLES OF APPLIED BEHAVIOR ANALYSIS

ABA is one intervention approach that provides a highly structured framework for learning. ABA is among the most extensively researched approaches to treat ASD, with established evidence for teaching specific skills to children with a range of disabilities. It is still important to understand that almost all of the evidence in support of ABA comes from single-subject designs rather than controlled group comparisons. This means that although ABA approaches do work for teaching skills, it is unknown whether they are better than other approaches because few systematic comparisons have been made.

ABA is based on a set of principles of learning that originated in the early 20th century. At the beginning of the 20th century, the Russian psychologist Ivan Pavlov published his work on what he called the "*conditioned reflex.*" Pavlov showed that dogs were able to produce a *reflexive behavior* (e.g., salivating) after begin exposed to a *stimulus* (e.g., a bell) that was consistently paired with a *reinforcer* (e.g., food). The dogs eventually salivated when they heard the bell even when food was not present. Pavlov's work demonstrated *classical conditioning,* or triggering an involuntary behavior with a specific stimulus through a process of learning. In the case of Pavlov's study, the matching of a neutral stimulus (the bell) with a reinforcer (food) produced the involuntary behavior (salivating) even without the reinforcer. The American psychologist John Watson was influenced by Pavlov's work and in 1913 published his "Behaviorist Manifesto," which

> ABA is among the most extensively researched approaches to treat ASD, with established evidence for teaching specific skills to children with a range of disabilities.

encouraged those interested in human psychology to focus on external behavior, rather than internal mental states.

The American psychologist B.F. Skinner (1965) built on Watson's foundation when he introduced what he called *behavior analysis* in the 1930s. Skinner was instrumental in bringing the ideas of behaviorism to the realm of education. He developed *"operant conditioning,"* or the modification of voluntary behavior (what he called *operant behavior*), as opposed to the *reflexive* behavior that Pavlov studied. In Skinner's view, operant behavior is behavior that is maintained by its consequences—a change in behavior is achieved through a large amount of repetition of desired actions, with rewards for these desired actions, along with discouragement for unwanted behaviors. *Positive reinforcement* (reward) and *negative reinforcement* (punishment) are the core tools of operant conditioning.

It was Ivar Lovaas who brought these ideas to the teaching of children with ASD. He reported the first demonstration of an effective way to teach children who are nonverbal to imitate, speak, and reduce self-injury and aggression. Lovaas's work also emphasized the importance of early and intensive intervention, parental involvement, and implementing interventions in natural settings, such as home and school, rather than hospitals or clinics. Although there are some issues about Lovaas's work—he may have made some unrealistic claims about the degree to which his methods succeeded—the important innovation he introduced was using teaching methods that were effective to some degree with children who were considered "unteachable." Whatever the result of the scientific debate about Lovaas's legacy, it is true that he introduced an important new tool for working with children with ASD, and generations of families of children with ASD have benefitted from this innovation.

One of the important contributions of ABA methods is the focus on specific, individual symptoms and behaviors rather than on general functioning. ABA methods can be used to teach specific skills such as pointing, saying words, using utensils to eat, or toilet training. ABA methods also can be used to reduce undesirable behaviors such as self-injury. It is crucial to understand that children treated with ABA still have autism, but can learn to show more adaptive behaviors and fewer maladaptive ones.

ABA has several advantages for children with ASD: 1) the majority of teaching is one to one; 2) it is highly structured to help children focus on the important information in the environment and pay attention to it and carefully designed to provide progress to goals in small, systematic steps; and 3) it is efficient in that it elicits a large number of target behaviors within each session so that the child has more opportunities to practice producing the desired behavior.

BEHAVIORAL PRINCIPLES: ANTECEDENT-BEHAVIOR-CONSEQUENCE

One basic idea behind the behaviorist approach is that *learning,* which behaviorists define as changing behavior, is accomplished through a large amount of repetition of desired actions. The way to get students to repeat these desired actions is by rewarding or reinforcing them. *Reinforcement* is defined as anything that increases a desired behavior. Although used less often with young children, punishment is another way to influence the behavior produced by the child. *Punishment* is defined as anything that reduces the frequency of an undesirable behavior. Teaching skills through ABA involves the ABCs.

> One basic idea behind the behaviorist approach is that *learning,* which behaviorists define as changing behavior, is accomplished through a large amount of repetition of desired actions.

- *A is for antecedent:* An antecedent is an event or feature in the environment that can affect behavior, also known as a *stimulus.* For example, a teacher clapping his or her hands in order to get the child to imitate is an antecedent. Showing a child a picture also can be an antecedent if the goal is to get the child to name the picture.

- *B is for behavior:* Behavior is an overt response produced to the antecedent. A child's clapping after the teacher's antecedent clapping is an example of a behavior; saying the name of the picture shown by the teacher is another example.

- *C is for consequence:* Consequence is the event that follows a behavior and affects the likelihood that the behavior will occur again in the future. A consequence can either be reinforcing or punishing. A *reinforcer* (e.g., a piece of candy) is a consequence that increases the likelihood that the behavior will occur again in the future. A *punishment* (e.g., taking away one of several tokens a child has been given) is a consequence that decreases the likelihood that the behavior will occur again in the future.

Many terms are used by behaviorists that are unfamiliar to people or are used in ways that are different from ordinary usage (see Table 7.1).

DISCRETE TRIAL INSTRUCTION

ABA is sometimes confused with discrete trial instruction (DTI). DTI is one of the many instructional strategies that are included in the broad ABA method, which is any teaching strategy that draws on behaviorist learning principles, including focusing on overt behavior, using consequences to influence the production of behavior, and assuming that behavior is controlled by consequences in the environment. DTI, however, is a particular type of ABA that is effective for teaching children with ASD because it provides a clear and simple framework for acquiring skills, especially skills that need to be practiced and memorized, such as learning the names of objects or learning a sequence of actions involved in a social-communication act like greeting. Each item or skill that is taught is broken down into a series of small steps in order to maximize the child's success. For example, when teaching a child to label an item such as a pen, the pen is shown to the child, the child is asked what it is using a specific phrase with the fewest

Table 7.1. Applied behavior analysis definitions for discrete trial instruction

Pairing/capturing child's attention	The first step in working with a child is for the adult to establish him- or herself as a reinforcer, sometimes referred to as pairing with the child. The adult observes the child at play, develops a list of potential reinforcers, and experiments with different reinforcers. Ideally, adults find reinforcers that can be controlled and can be paired with words, (e.g., tickles, bubbles, books). Once the reinforcers are identified, the adult pairs him- or herself with them. The adult needs to be in control of reinforcer delivery so that the child has access to reinforcers through the adult and therefore associates interaction with the adult with fun things.
Setting-Antecedent-Behavior-Consequence (SABC) model	This four-term contingency used for discrete trial instruction and behavior analysis consists of a setting (S), antecedent (A), behavior (B), and consequence (C). For example, the setting is that the bell has rung when it is time to leave the playground and go inside.
Prompting and fading prompts	Prompting is an action to help the child correctly respond while performing discrete trials. Following are the different prompts, ranging from the most intrusive to the least intrusive: 1. Physical prompt 2. Partial physical prompt 3. Imitative prompt 4. Gestural prompt 5. Echoic prompt and partial echoic prompt 6. Position prompt 7. Direct verbal prompt 8. Indirect verbal prompt Always use the least intrusive prompt that will lead to success because it will make fading prompts easier.
Fading	Fading is the systematic withdrawal of prompting when teaching a specific behavior so that prompts are more subtle over time. To keep motivation high, reinforcement is adjusted so that the more independent the response is, the greater the reinforcement (value).
Managing/understanding consequences	The tendency for a behavior to occur again in the future depends on the consequence that follows the behavior. A reinforcer is a consequence that increases the likelihood that the behavior will occur again in the future. A punisher (i.e., ignoring or removing an item) is a consequence that decreases the likelihood that the behavior will occur again in the future.
Errorless learning	Errorless learning occurs when the instruction is presented in such a way that the possibility of an incorrect response is minimal.
Shaping	Shaping is used when the response required is too complex to occur, even with a correction procedure. The adult gradually reinforces responses that are close to the required behavior (e.g., an approximation of the sign is accepted until it eventually resembles the target sign). There are three elements to the shaping procedure: 1. Target response 2. Starting point 3. Successive approximations
Chaining	Chaining is the linking of discrete behaviors into a more complex, composite behavior. Chaining is useful for teaching behaviors that occur essentially in the same order each time and is especially useful for teaching self-help skills such as washing hands or brushing teeth.
Task analysis	A task analysis is breaking down a behavior into its component behaviors. Daily routines such as washing hands or brushing teeth are comprised of a series of distinct simple behaviors performed one after another.

possible words (e.g., "What is it?"), the adult provides the necessary supports and prompts for response (e.g., telling the child, "It's a pen. You say pen"), and reinforces, or rewards, the correct response, or provides feedback and correction. See Figure 7.1 for an example of a discrete trial.

Mixing material the child already knows with new material the child is still learning is another feature of DTI. The ratio of known to unknown material is 80%:20% when first starting intervention in order to maintain the child's motivation. The ratio changes to 50:50 as the child progresses. The child is still spending some time reviewing material that has already been learned and some time learning new responses.

*A*BA is sometimes confused with discrete trial instruction (DTI). DTI is one of the many instructional strategies that are included in the broad ABA method, which is any teaching strategy that draws on behaviorist learning principles.

DTI takes advantage of *shaping,* which is a basic technique of behavioral instruction. How are you going to teach a child to say "cookie" in order to get a cookie, if the child can't say "cookie?" The behaviorist's answer is shaping. The child is rewarded for producing an *approximation,* or getting close to the target behavior, in the early stages of teaching. If the child can't say "cookie," then any vocal output might be rewarded with a cookie at first. Once the child consistently makes a sound for the cookie, the interventionist requires progressively closer approximations in order to get the reward. First, the child might have to say "oo" to get the cookie, then "koo," then "kook," then finally "cookie." Part of the art of this kind of intervention is in knowing what to accept as an approximation, for how long, when to require more, and so forth.

There are several advantages to DTI methods. First, it is easy to keep specific data on progress within a DTI framework. Figure 7.2 provides an example of the kind of data sheet a therapist might use. Multiple instructors can work with the child because the skill taught— expected behavior—as well as level of mastery is always recorded. This is advantageous especially when a team of adults are involved in working with one child. In summary, the advantages of using DTI include

A DISCRETE TRIAL INVOLVES THREE STEPS:

Example of a discrete trial

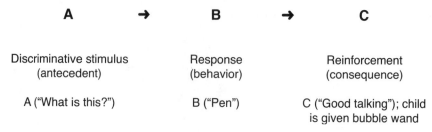

A	→	B	→	C
Discriminative stimulus (antecedent)		Response (behavior)		Reinforcement (consequence)
A ("What is this?")		B ("Pen")		C ("Good talking"); child is given bubble wand

Figure 7.1. Example of a discrete trial.

- The correct response is clear to instructor and student.

- It allows many trials in a short time, so there is a lot of practice.

- Different instructors can consistently use the same method.

- Data recording is simple.

Although DTI can theoretically be used to teach any skill, communication is one of the primary impairments in ASD, and there are several programs specifically designed to teach spoken communication to children that primarily make use of a DTI format. *The Me Book* is Lovaas's (1981) manual for using DTI to teach language to children with ASD. *Teach Me Language,* developed by Freeman, Dake, and Davis (1996), the Assessment of Basic Language and Learning Skills (ABLLS-R) developed by Partington and Sundberg (1998), and Verbal Behavior–Milestones Assessment and Placement Program (VB-MAPP), (VB-MAPP; Sundberg, 2008), are three other DTI programs for teaching communication skills. The VB-MAPP and ABLLS-R program have a sizeable amount of single-subject and multiple-baseline research to support them.

Rethink Autism (http://www.rethinkautism.com) is another program that takes advantage of DTI methodology. This web-based curriculum provides on-line videos of carefully sequenced DTI activities that can be used to help parents and educators create and deliver an educational program for a child with ASD. The videos serve as models for instruction. Assessment tools provided as part of the program allow educators to identify the child's current level of functioning, choose the most appropriate next steps in the curricular sequence, and use the video models as a guide to providing the individualized instruction. Although no research has been reported on the web-based curriculum, the basic principles of DTI that it uses to construct the program have a well-established research base.

NATURALISTIC APPLIED BEHAVIOR ANALYSIS METHODS OF INSTRUCTION

There are some disadvantages to the DTI approach. One is that children can become too dependent on the prompts and rewards provided by the therapist. They may become passive and fail to initiate any actions or interactions. They may not comply with instructions if they aren't continually and explicitly rewarded. The second disadvantage is that children can succeed at very high levels in the DTI format, but fail to carry the skills over into real-world situations. They may perform 90% correct on naming pictures in the therapy setting, for example, but be unable to name the objects the pictures represent when they see them in a different setting. ABA practitioners became keenly aware of these

> Children can succeed at very high levels in the DTI format but fail to carry the skills over into real-world situations. They may perform 90% correct on naming pictures in the therapy setting, for example, but be unable to name the objects the pictures represent when they see them in a different setting.

Session: Gross motor imitation

DATE: 3/13/2015 _____ DISCRIMINATIVE STIMULUS (SD): Do this _____

Description						
	3/13	3/14	3/15	3/16	3/17	3/18
1. Clap hands	3	2	+	+	+	A
2. Arms up	2	1	+	+	+	A
3. Tap knees	1	1	+	+	+	A
4. Touch nose	1	1	+	+	+	A
5.						
6.						
7.						
8.						
9.						
10.						
11.						
12.						
13.						
14.						
15.						

+ Achieved 1 Imitative Prompt 2 Partial physical prompt 3 Hand over hand prompt	Prompts: Gestures Indirect verbal prompt Single verbal prompt Multiple verbal prompt Imitative prompt Physical prompt Hand over hand

Figure 7.2. Sample data sheet. (*Key:* + = independent; 1 = imitative prompt; 2 = physical; 3 = hand over hand; A = achieved)

disadvantages as they worked with their students and began to develop strategies to combat them. As a result, ABA intervention looks very different today than it did when Lovaas was doing his work in the 1970s. Researchers and therapists alike have come to recognize the importance of integrating newly learned skills into daily routines and functional activities and reducing the child's dependence on antecedent prompts to elicit functional behaviors and on tangible rewards to maintain them. ABA theorists have developed a range of tactics to address these shortcomings, and including these alternate approaches in a comprehensive intervention program is advocated by all reputable ABA therapists today. ABA programs can vary with regard to the balance of activities they use; some parts of the day may be focused on DTI, whereas others include activities that look more like play or less structured teaching. These activities are usually called *naturalistic ABA* because they maintain certain principles of the behaviorist philosophy, even though they may look as if the child is just playing in a natural way to the untrained eye.

The major innovation of naturalistic behavior programs is that instead of using the ABC sequence (Antecedent [educator says, "Say cookie"]-Behavior [child says, "Cookie"]-Consequence [educator gives the child a cookie]), the instruction follows the child's behavior. The sequence is as follows in naturalistic ABA:

- Behavior (emitted by child: reaches for cookie in closed jar)

- Instruction (presented by educator: "Oh, you want the cookie! Say, 'Cookie.'" Instructor waits for child to say "cookie" or something close)

- Response (child gives approximation of "cookie")

- Consequence (instructor opens the jar and gives child cookie)

Educators using naturalistic ABA engineer the environment so things the child will want require some adult assistance; they may put goodies in containers the child can't open or on high shelves that are hard to reach or hide important parts of a toy or game where the child can't see them. They then wait for the child to show interest in something (this first move on the child's part is key because it helps the child learn to initiate an interaction instead of waiting for a prompt, or antecedent) and only provide access to these things when the child follows an instruction with an appropriate response. Other key features of naturalistic ABA include the following:

> Educators using naturalistic ABA engineer the environment so things the child will want require some adult assistance

- The educator chooses objects and activities and "plants" them in the environment.

- Instruction takes place in the context of natural activities using objects of high interest to the child.

- The child selects the stimulus to focus on from a set provided by the educator, so the child has some control over the content of the session.

- The educator gives prompts based on the child's initiating behavior, rather than a predetermined order of presentation.

- Instruction may take place on the floor, rather than at a table; more child movement and choice is accepted.

There are quite a few brands of naturalistic behavioral intervention, those that focus on specific behaviors and those that are more comprehensive approaches. The ones mentioned here are those that have reported some outcomes in the research literature (see Table 6.1 on page 153 and Table 6.2 on page 155). Other comprehensive programs or targeted interventions may also work, but published research is not currently available to evaluate them and, therefore, they are not included in this section. Let's look at some of the comprehensive programs designed to provide generalized curricula for young children with ASD.

COMPREHENSIVE PROGRAMS TO ADDRESS ASD SYMPTOMS

Programs like those in Table 6.1 are designed to address the full range of needs of children with ASD, as outlined in the The National Research Council's (2001) report. The discussion of comprehensive programs here is divided into the three categories previously mentioned based on their underlying assumptions about learning—*ABA methods, developmental/pragmatic programs,* and *relationship-based programs.* The guiding principles associated with each of these are discussed in their respective sections.

Naturalistic Applied Behavior Analysis Programs

The naturalistic ABA approach has been applied in a range of comprehensive programs designed to provide a complete educational curriculum for children with ASD. These programs generally are delivered in specialized preschool and school settings. The comprehensive programs that have reported some evidence regarding their outcomes include the Treatment and Education of Autistic and related Communication Handicapped Children (TEACCH) method (Schopler et al., 2004), Pivotal Response Training (PRT; Koegel & Koegel, 2006), the Douglass Developmental Disabilities Center (Harris et al., 2000), the Learning Experiences and Alternative Program (LEAP) preschool (Strain & Bovey, 2011), the Princeton Child Development Institute (Fenske et al., 1985), and the Strategies for Teaching based on Autism Research (STAR) program (Arick et al., 2003). These are listed in Table 6.1 on page 153. Some of these are site specific; that is, they are available only in the limited geographic area covered by the facility that houses them. Others, such as PRT (http://www.autismprthelp.com/) provide training services beyond their own site. Table 7.2 provides examples of some of the procedures from just one of these programs, PRT, to give you a sense of what they look like.

Table 7.2. Examples of pivotal response behaviors

Pivotal behavior	Rationale	Methods	Examples
Responding to multiple cues	Increases generalization from one object to classes of objects	*Within stimulus prompting:* exaggerating features of a stimulus, then gradually fading the exaggerations *Conditional discriminations:* requiring discrimination on the basis of more than one feature	When teaching the sign for MORE, the sign is first demonstrated with large sweeping arm motions and exaggerated closing of the hands, which are gradually faded. When teaching colors, the child is asked to get a blue sock and is presented with a blue sock, a white sock, and a blue shirt so that he or she must consider both the color and the item name in making a choice.
Increasing motivation	Increases responsiveness to the social environment and enhance spontaneity and generalization	*Child choice:* let the child select preferred games, topics, toys, and activities within teaching situations *Natural reinforcers:* give rewards that are directly related to the activity *Interspersing maintenance trails:* include practice of activities already learned to give child a sense of success *Reinforcing attempts:* use shaping to reward any goal-directed behavior, even if it is not the direct target	When teaching colors, child is allowed to choose colored candies. When teaching *cup,* the child is given a cup with juice in it after he or she names the object. Teaching a new skill is preceded by several trials of a well-learned skill that has a high probability of being performed correctly. When teaching a pointing gesture as a request, a fist point is rewarded if it clearly indicates communication, then it is shaped by gradually increasing requirement for index finger isolation.
Increasing self-regulation	Improves independence; provides more opportunities for spontaneous social interaction without supervision	*Target behaviors are operationally defined:* child has clear idea of what to do *Reinforcers are identified:* rewarding consequences are used *Self-monitoring is selected, trained, and validated:* a simple method of tracking child's own behavior is provided	Through repeated modeling, the child is taught to touch a teacher's arm whenever peer moves too close to him or her for comfort. Child is rewarded for alerting the teacher rather than pushing peer by being allowed to play a favorite music box. Child gets a star and puts it on his or her hand each time he or she alerts the teacher rather than pushing peer. Teacher checks child's hand after free play period and provides praise for the number of stars he or she earned.
Increasing initiation of communication	Increase opportunities for spontaneous social learning and increased social competence	*Motivation to communicate is built into activities* *Prompt/fade and shaping techniques are used to support initiations*	Preferred objects are placed in an opaque bag. Child is prompted to ask, "What's that?" Child is allowed to play with toy after asking question. Prompts are gradually faded.

Sources: Koegel, Koegel, Harrower, and Carter (1999); Paul and Sutherland (2005).

Another comprehensive ABA program not included in Table 6.1 is Natural Environment Training (NET), developed in the late 1990s by James Partington and Mark Sundberg. Although it does not have published outcome data as a comprehensive program, NET is an extension of the VB-MAPP approach, which does show published evidence of efficacy. NET places emphasis on building rapport with the child and using this rapport, along with the provision of desired objects and activities, to accomplish intervention goals. This process of building motivation through connection is referred to as *pairing* in NET. By pairing or connecting with the child, the adult becomes a reinforcer by being seen as a valued play partner, someone with whom the child wants to engage. NET requires observing the child across a variety of settings and identifying items and activities that the child finds rewarding and enjoyable. NET starts with the adult in control of reinforcers so that the child associates fun and excitement with the adult. The pairing concept encourages the addition of social reinforcers, such as tickling or singing, and includes verbal foreshadowing of rewards with statements such as, "Here comes a tickle!" or "Here come the bubbles!"

The NET method also focuses on the importance of avoiding negative pairing or adverse associations with the adult. For example, if a child is seated on the floor having fun looking at a book or playing with playdough, then rather than interrupting the fun activity with a demand, NET therapists first join in and introduce an activity that is even more fun. Once pairing is achieved, simple demands that are easy to comply with can be made, such as asking the child to do something he or she was about to do anyway, or has often done before, followed by reinforcing the compliance. The child eventually comes to associate reinforcement with compliance and will be motivated to comply with additional, more demanding instructions. Table 7.3 provides examples of pairing procedures.

A large, systematic review of comprehensive ABA-based programs for young children with ASD by Magiati, Wei, and Howlin (2012) found that early comprehensive naturalistic behavioral interventions resulted in improved outcomes, particularly in cognitive functioning, with smaller gains in language and adaptive behavior. Moreover, their review found that these early, intensive, behaviorally based comprehensive approaches, which involve 15–25 hours of intervention per week, highly trained and supervised personnel, and carefully prescribed

Table 7.3.   The do's and don'ts of pairing

Do's	Don'ts
Join in child-initiated activities	Make demands
Provide tangible rewards	Reinforce inappropriate behavior
Verbally praise	Interrupt pairing with questions
Be sincere	Leave reinforcers out
Offer choice and control delivery of reinforcers	
Pair self with reinforcement	
Observe child's willingness to interact with you	

assessment and treatment procedures detailed in program manuals written by university-based program developers, are "more likely to lead to better intellectual, language and/or adaptive behavioral outcomes compared with nonspecific 'eclectic' provisions or other, less intensive interventions" (p. 546). Magiati and colleagues noted though that the various comprehensive approaches have been compared only with less intensive, less systematic community treatments and not to each other to determine which are most effective or which elements of the program work best. Samuel Odom and his colleagues (Odom, Boyd, et al., 2010; and Odom, Collet-Klinterberg, et al., 2010) also reviewed a range of comprehensive programs and evaluated their characteristics. Their review is incorporated in the information presented in Tables 6.1 and 6.2.

Developmental/Pragmatic Approaches

Developmental/pragmatic (D/P) approaches make a different set of assumptions about learning than ABA methods. ABA theory holds that behavior is controlled by consequences in the environment and learning takes place when these consequences are systematically manipulated to elicit, stabilize, and maintain desired behavior. D/P approaches, however, emphasize the role of the natural interactions and social motivation in guiding the normal sequence of typical development. These approaches focus on functional communication, the use of a variety of strategies, such as gestures, gaze, and vocalizations in addition to language to send meaningful messages to others. They are primarily concerned with providing the child with a developmentally appropriate way to get wants and needs across and to provide opportunities for the child to develop and express a range of different communicative functions. An ABA therapist may teach requests first as sounds, then as single words, then as two-word utterances, and then as sentences. A D/P therapist, however, might move from requests as soon as they are acquired to teaching different functions of communication, such as pointing things out to people and rejecting unwanted activities, even if the forms used to express these remain at the single-word or even gestural level. Although an ABA therapist might try to *extinguish* (get rid of) vocal and gestural communication, or even echolalia once a child started talking, D/P approaches encourage the use of multiple channels of communication even after the child starts using words.

Developmental/pragmatic (D/P) approaches make a different set of assumptions about learning than ABA methods. ABA theory holds that behavior is controlled by consequences in the environment and learning takes place when these consequences are systematically manipulated to elicit, stabilize, and maintain desired behavior. D/P approaches, however, emphasize the role of the natural interactions and social motivation in guiding the normal sequence of typical development.

Finally, whereas ABA therapists would use shaping to mold early communicative behaviors into more appropriate forms, D/P therapists would first respond to anything a child does and treat it as if it were communicative, even if the child didn't really intend it that way. For example, rather than trying to elicit some communicative behavior from a nonverbal child, a D/P therapist might use play with some of the child's preferred toys, and respond any time the child touched a toy as if the child were pointing at it and asking for its name, even if the child gave no indication of wanting to hear the label or directing the act to the therapist.

D/P approaches assume that the normal sequence of communicative development provides the best guidelines for determining intervention goals. These approaches aim to provide intensified opportunities for children with ASD to have the same communication experiences that typically developing peers have, in the belief that these are the most effective (because they are the most natural) contexts for learning social-communication skills. D/P therapy takes advantage of learning opportunities ("teachable moments") that naturally arise in the course of interactions, rather than relying on a predetermined curriculum. Therapists aim to provide facilitating interactions, which are defined as

- Focusing on what a child is already interested in; acknowledging and responding to the child's intent, even if it is not expressed through speech

- Modeling ways to communicate about activities in which the child is already engaged

- Expanding on what the child spontaneously produces

- Targeting behaviors that can be used in daily, meaningful activities in a variety of situations apart from the therapy setting in which they were originally learned

- Assuming the prerequisite role of nonverbal communication, including gestures, gaze, vocalization, and other nonvocal means, in the development of language so that speech is not the first target for children who are nonverbal; instead, the expression of communication through these other means is encouraged

Another assumption of the D/P approach is that children with ASD develop language in the same way and following the same sequence as typically developing children. This means that children who are nonverbal will first be encouraged to use other means of communicating to get ideas across in order to learn about the value of communication, as children with typical development do in the transition from preverbal to verbal communication (at about 12–24 months of age). Proponents of this approach advocate the use of a variety of nonverbal forms of communication as a stepping stone to speech.

The Early Start Denver Model (Rogers & Dawson, 2010) is one D/P program that has a high level of evidence (Table 6.1 provides a link to the program). One study of this program is a randomized controlled design, and a detailed manual is available that facilitates the use of the program in community settings. The Social Communication, Emotional Regulation, Transactional Support (SCERTS®)

program (Prizant, Wetherby, Rubin, Laurent, & Rydell, 2006) is another comprehensive D/P program, but it has little in the way of empirical support as of this writing.

Relationship-Based Therapy

Relationship-based approaches take the position that what children with ASD need is not so much to learn specific skills as to develop meaningful relationships with others that will make them want to learn new skills in order to enhance these interactions. Relationship-based approaches assume that what drives learning is not so much the desire for an external, tangible reward but the satisfaction that comes from connecting with others.

It might occur to you that the flaw in this reasoning is that children with ASD are lacking the ability to derive positive feelings from engaging with others, but relationship-based approaches make the assumption that this feeling can be fostered if adults make themselves the source of experiences the child with ASD enjoys, even though these experiences are different from what other children find enjoyable. For example, many children with ASD enjoy spinning objects, which is not particularly appealing for typically developing children for very long. ABA therapists might engineer the environment to exclude items that the child could get overly focused on spinning and only provide toys, such as blocks, that can be used more adaptively. A relationship-based intervention approach, however, might allow the child to have items that can spin, allow a brief period of spinning, then playfully interrupt it by putting a hand over the object and waiting for the child to look at the adult to see what the problem is. The adult might ask to take a turn spinning, make a remark such as, "Spinning is fun," or help the child get the object spinning again. This sequence may be repeated until the child begins to anticipate the adult's action and even to look forward to it. Enhancing the enjoyment of interaction is the goal of these activities. The adult would not insist on any particular response because building a positive relationship, rather than producing a particular behavior, is considered important in a relationship-based program. These programs tend to be comprehensive in nature because the focus on relationship building makes them less likely to identify specific skills to target. Relationship Development Intervention (RDI) and Floortime are two well-known programs that take a relationship-based approach.

> Enhancing the enjoyment of interaction is the goal of these activities.
>
> Building a positive relationship, rather than producing a particular behavior, is considered important in a relationship-based program.

Relationship Development Intervention   RDI is a trademarked, proprietary treatment developed by Steven Gutstein (Gutstein et al., 2002). Parents and teachers must pay fees to its originators for training in order to use the treatment.

The treatment is primarily family based, with consultants provided to teach family members how to provide the child with guided participation in relationships. Activities are aimed at building motivation and skills for successfully interacting in these relationships. The activities used in the program often are fun and motivating to many children with ASD. Like other relationship-based programs, they focus on creating opportunities for the child to enjoy being with others, rather than on teaching specific skills. The authors have published two studies without any comparison groups, and no independent studies have been published. Therefore, this treatment is considered to show emerging rather than established efficacy.

Developmental, Individual Difference, Relationship-based/Floortime Program

The Developmental, Individual Difference, Relationship-based (DIR) program also is a trademarked and proprietary system developed by Greenspan & Wieder (1998). The developmental aspect of the program is aimed at fostering capacities considered by the program creators to be the basic milestones of early development, including attending, relating, purposefully communicating, problem solving, using ideas creatively, and using ideas logically. The individual differences component of the program focuses on the ways each particular child understands sensations, such as sound and touch, and tries to find ways to accommodate each child's sensitivities to these stimuli. The relationship-based element aims to help adults tailor their interactions to the child's individual differences and developmental capacities. Activities are designed not only to follow the child's natural interests, but also to challenge the child during these playful interactions that occur in naturalistic settings, which often occur while sitting on the floor (hence, Floortime). Adults are encouraged first to join in any activity the child is enjoying, whether playing with toys, spinning objects, or repeatedly turning a light switch off and on. Once the child understands that the adult is willing to share favorite activities, adults are taught to use playful obstruction strategies to create opportunities for the child to engage in interactions through the shared activity. For example, if an adult is playing with a child and a favorite toy, then the adult might hide the toy outside the door, show it to the child, and then close the door. When the child bangs on the door, the adult can ask, "Shall I help you?" then provide the toy. The child is expected to provide more spontaneous and complex communications within this relationship over time. Like RDI, the DIR authors provide a few small case studies without contrast groups or controls, so the evidence in support of this approach is considered emerging rather than established.

In summary, comprehensive intervention programs that derive from each of the three philosophical approaches to intervention for ASD have been developed. As such, there is a fairly wide variety of programs available. At this time, the comprehensive approaches with the strongest evidence base are drawn from the naturalistic behavioral model.

TARGETED, SPECIFIC INTERVENTION TECHNIQUES WITH AN EVIDENCE BASE

Although comprehensive programs aim to address a range of aspects and symptoms of ASD, targeted interventions are designed to address specific behaviors and are incorporated with other techniques. Targeted interventions do not comprise a program on their own, but instead are aimed to change a small set of behaviors. Table 6.2 on page 155 lists a wide range of these specific practices that have been shown to have some degree of evidence for being helpful in teaching new skills to children with ASD. The focus here is on a few techniques that have shown efficacy for improving social-communication skills in young children with ASD.

Naturalistic Behavioral Techniques

Like comprehensive programs derived from the naturalistic behavioral model, there is a relatively large set of specific intervention techniques that are drawn from naturalistic ABA. We will describe a sampling of them here, mostly those focused on the development of social communication skills.

Milieu or Incidental Teaching   This method goes by a variety of names, including milieu communication training, incidental teaching, and mand-modeling. The methods primarily focus on developing communication skills and are integrated into a child's natural environment. They have a relatively strong, although still emerging, basis in evidence from both case studies and group designs. Milieu teaching strategies include

- Training in everyday environments (e.g., home, classroom), rather than a therapy room

- Providing activities that take place throughout the day, rather than only at therapy time

- Engineering the environment so that preferred toys and activities are in sight but out of reach so children require adult assistance in order to get items they want

- Encouraging spontaneous communication by refraining from prompting and using *expectant waiting* (use of gaze, posture, and facial expression to indicate the adult expects the child to do something)

- Allowing the child to initiate a teaching situation by means of a gesture or by indicating interest in a desired object or activity

- Allowing teachers to provide prompts and cues for expanding the child's initiation

- Rewarding expanded child responses with access to a desired object or activity

Examples of milieu teaching approaches appear in Table 7.4.

Table 7.4.   Examples of milieu teaching strategies

Method	Example activity
Prompt free	Pictures of toys or snacks are placed within a child's reach. When the child touches one of the pictures (whether intentionally or not), the child is given the object pictured. This continues until the child intentionally and spontaneously uses the pictures to request desired objects.
Mand-model approach	Objects the child likes are placed in sight but out of reach. The teacher observes the child and when interest is shown in an object, even fleeting interest, the teacher "mands" (requests) an utterance from the child with a stimulus such as, "What's that?" If the child responds with the target word or gesture, then he or she receives the toy to play with for a short time. It is later replaced so it can tempt the child.
Milieu communication training	Objects the child likes are placed in sight but out of reach around the classroom. The teacher waits for the child to indicate interest in an object by looking at it or pulling an adult toward it. When the child does, the teacher uses expectant waiting to allow the child to initiate a request. If a conventional request is not produced, then the teacher prompts with, "What do you want?" If the child produces the target response (pointing to or naming the object), then he or she receives the desired object to play with for a time. It is later replaced to be used again. If the child does not produce the target, then the teacher provides a fuller prompt, such as request for direct imitation of the target ("You want the bear? Say, 'bear.'") and receives the toy.

Sources: Hart and Risley (1975); Mirenda and Santogrossi (1985); Paul and Sutherland (2005); Rogers-Warren and Warren (1980).

Responsive education and prelinguistic milieu teaching (RPMT) is one variant of milieu teaching that also has some supportive emerging evidence. RPMT involves providing therapist-delivered intervention using milieu teaching techniques to children who are nonverbal, with the aim of encouraging first gestural and vocal communication and eventually words. Crucially, it also includes training for parents to provide high levels of responsiveness, defined as using milieu teaching techniques in their own day-to-day interactions with their children. Again, several studies have documented emerging evidence for improving communication and speech with this approach.

Script Fading

Many children with ASD engage in *scripting* when they start to talk; they may repeat television commercials or portions of movies they've seen, often to themselves without any apparent communicative intent. McClannahan and Krantz (2005) developed a method that uses this tendency to script to improve communication skills in children with ASD at a wide range of developmental levels. A script for preschoolers might include a set of audio-recorded words, phrases, or sentences that the child listens to and repeats. Alternatively, a script may be a set of picture cards, each of which is associated with a word or gesture, and the child is taught through behavioral techniques to produce the script in response to the pictures in an appropriate social situation. Scripts for older children often are written on a sequenced set of cue cards. Once the script has been repeatedly practiced, the cue card or audio is faded by deleting one portion at a time until the child independently produces the entire script. This method has been demonstrated to be effective in a range of single case studies. Comic strip conversations use a similar approach, employing comic strips rather than written scripts (Gray, 1994).

Developmental/Pragmatic Techniques

D/P approaches also have been developed for specific skill targets. Again, we focus here on those aimed primarily at social communication goals.

More Than Words   More Than Words was derived from approaches developed by The Hanen Centre for training parents and teachers to facilitate language development by providing enriched, contingent, and stimulating input to children with a range of disabilities. Training parents and teachers of preschool children with ASD to promote social-communication skills within ordinary interactions throughout the child's day is the focus of More Than Words, the Hanen approach to autism. Some elements common to the activities found in More Than Words, as well as in other D/P intervention approaches, include the following.

- Following the child's lead by noticing what the child is doing and then joining in, even if the child attempts to refuse the adult's intrusion

- Treating any behavior as if it were communicative (if the child is playing with the parent's keys, then this behavior can be treated as if it were a request to ride in the car and take the child for a ride, or pretend to)

- Imitating the child's sounds and actions, rather than asking the child to imitate the adult

- Turning the child's preferred activities into games (e.g., if the child likes to roll cars back and forth, parents can initiate a car race by intruding and imitating)

- Modeling and encouraging turn taking in a variety of sound and action games

- Using visual supports (See Figures 7.3, 7.4, and 7.5), such as picture cue cards, visual schedules, picture stories, and computer games

- Using music to support attention to language by embedding simple language in short, slowly produced song formats with heavy stress placed on important words

A few small studies have examined the outcomes of More Than Words intervention at this time, and the evidence for it is considered emerging.

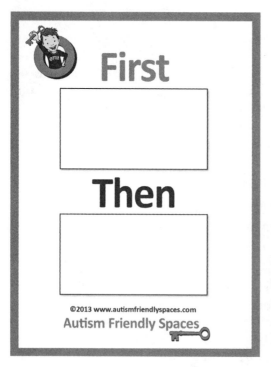

Figure 7.3. Example of a visual support for sequencing.

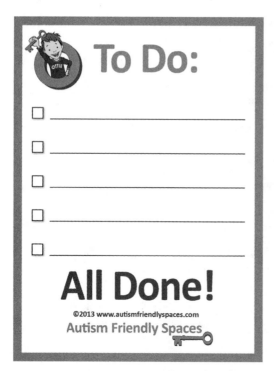

Figure 7.4. Example of a visual support for task completion.

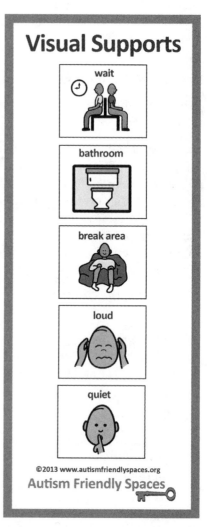

Figure 7.5. Example of visual supports for classroom participation.

Social Narratives

This approach uses stories written in collaboration with children to outline and structure social interactions, particularly those that can be problematic for a particular child. The stories usually are illustrated with simple drawings and repeatedly read with the child, similar to reading a favorite picture book. Once the child has memorized the text of the story, it can be recalled and used as self-talk, with coaching from the therapist, in real situations with peers. Figure 7.6 gives an example of a social narrative that might be used with an older preschool or young school-age child. There also are commercially available versions, such as Gray and Attwood's (2010) *New Social Stories Book—Revised and Expanded,* as well as social story apps for electronic platforms, such as *Social Story Creator* by Touch Autism. Additional story creation apps are available at TinyTap (http://www.tinytap.it/).

Joint Attention

The ability to share attention with others and the capacity to engage in pretend play are considered important, pivotal skills for communication and learning. Joint attention serves as a basis both for developing language—because children need to focus on what others point out in order to get the connection between the words they use and the things they attend to—and for developing interactive play—because playing with others requires attending to the objects and activities they choose. Teaching children to share attention to objects with therapists, and eventually rewarding children for directing the therapist's attention to objects and activities, has been examined by several researchers, including Kasari et al., (2008). Their findings provide established evidence that focusing on joint attention is helpful in improving social interaction and spoken language outcomes.

Symbolic Play

Most children with ASD have difficulty not only with joint attention but also with the ability to pretend or use symbolic play. In fact, the lack of imaginative play was considered one of the diagnostic criteria for autism for some years, although it is no longer listed as a primary symptom in the *DSM-5* (2013). The ability to pretend, to let a stick stand for a gun or a block for a car, is not just for fun. It allows the child to practice using *representational thought*, or to hold an idea in mind and impose the idea on playthings, using them as *symbols,* to represent something other than what they really are. As we saw in Chapter 2, young children's use of symbolic play gives them the opportunity to engage this symbolic function of the mind, which is the basis for language and other kinds of abstract mental activity. Language is particularly related to symbolic development because words are used to represent the objects and ideas they refer to. It allows speakers to cause listeners to form mental pictures of objects referred

My name is Frankie.
I have friends at school.

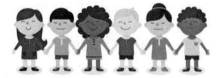

Sometimes my friends like to play my favorite games.

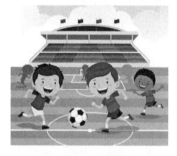

Sometimes my friends don't want to play my favorite games.

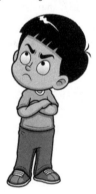

This is because we all like to do different things.

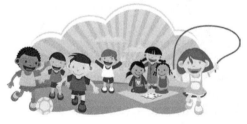

I can get upset and sad when this happens.

I will try to play their games more so that I will have somebody to play with.

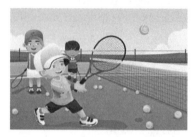

This will help me because my friends will see that I am trying to share and be a kind person.

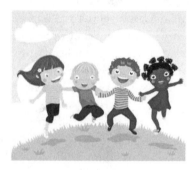

This will make me happy and my friends and my teacher happy.

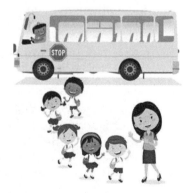

Figure 7.6. Example of a social narrative.

to, by means of the exchange of the word that stands for it. Even children with language delays not associated with ASD tend to have reduced levels of pretend play, and the two abilities seem to develop in tandem, at least in the early stages of language acquisition.

It stands to reason, then, that if a child has difficulty with both language and symbolic play, as children with ASD as well as other language problems often do, then encouraging both pretending and communicating with words could strengthen both capacities. Teaching symbolic play—through modeling, imitating, reinforcing attempts, and providing a lot of fun consequences when a child uses an object for a pretend purpose—has established evidence of improving both social and language skills in children with ASD. Kasari's group (2008, 2014) has combined teaching joint attention and play skills in their joint attention and symbolic play engagement regulation (JASPER) technique to good effect in young children with ASD.

VISUAL SUPPORTS

Children with autism often seem more comfortable with information that is presented visually, rather than in the form of sound (see Chapter 2). Visual supports can be either written (if the child can read) or pictorial representations of a series of activities in which they are expected to participate, and are often used with this population. Teachers and therapists may develop their own visual supports, such as visual schedules that depict a series of actions that need to be followed or the sequence of events, activities, transitions, or times of the day that prove difficult for the child with ASD to get through. Figures 7.3–7.5 provide some examples of these kinds of supports. Computer programs and tablet apps allow users to generate visual schedules, checklists, and so forth using clip art, text, and photographs that users can put into the system to personalize the material. These forms of visual support are considered to have established evidence of helping children with ASD understand and manage classroom and other social situations.

AUGMENTATIVE AND ALTERNATIVE COMMUNICATION

Many therapists believe that if a child does not talk, then it is important to foster some way to express wants and needs, even if only temporarily until speech emerges, by supplying a nonoral, nonvocal way to communicate in the form of signs, pictures, or an electronic device. Parents often worry that introducing AAC means the therapist is giving up on teaching the child to speak. Although it is important to continue to devote some degree of attention to encouraging vocal and verbal communication in young children with ASD, providing an AAC mode can help a child overcome frustration at being unable to get meaning across in the present circumstance. Several techniques are designed to provide children with this more accessible way of communicating.

Picture Exchange Communication System

PECS is an AAC system designed for children who have not developed any spoken language. PECS has a lot of single case study and group comparison research, suggesting it does provide improvement in communication for children with ASD who are nonverbal and is considered a method with established evidence. A PECS program begins with teaching single-word requests by means of exchanging a picture for an object. Like naturalistic ABA approaches, PECS focuses on child initiation of communicative acts. It requires the child to begin an exchange by handing a picture to an adult in order to obtain the pictured object. Direct verbal prompts such as, "What do you want?" are avoided to help increase the spontaneity of requests. A favorite reinforcer is identified at the start of the training, and a picture of it is put in front of the child while an adult holds up the desired object out of the child's reach. A second adult sits behind the child and guides the child's hand to pick up the picture and give it to the first adult, in exchange for the object. Spontaneity and generalization of the picture exchanges are introduced by

- Fading the second adult's guidance once the child begins spontaneously initiating the exchanges

- Gradually increasing the distance between the child and the pictures

- Using the system in different environments

- Involving a variety of people

Two pictures are offered once the child can independently exchange one picture, and the child must choose the picture that matches the object held by the adult in order to complete the exchange. The program continues to increase the complexity of tasks by providing more picture choices, expanding from requests to labels and descriptions and eventually requiring the child to string several picture symbols together ("I" + "want" + "cookie;" "I" + "see" + "brown" + "bear").

Other Augmentative and Alternative Communication Approaches

Signs used by deaf communicators have been used for many years to provide a communication system for children with ASD who are nonverbal. Although some children with ASD do learn a few signs, which can be helpful in expressing basic needs, evidence suggests they do not evolve past single signs to fully functional communication systems as they do in children who are deaf.

Many AAC approaches are going beyond signs and pictures to using electronic devices, particularly smartphones and tablet computers, to supply portable, easily accessible means of providing those who are nonverbal with a large range of images, text, and the ability to turn typing into digitized or synthetic speech. Many functions that were previously supplied by expensive, dedicated AAC devices can now be found on consumer electronic platforms such as iPads. These voice output communication aids (VOCAs) are not only cheaper and easier to use, but also, because they use mobile devices platforms that are familiar and less stigmatizing are likely to increase peers' enthusiasm for interacting with the user with ASD. Several apps are available and range in price from $24.99 to $249.99. My Very First AAC, at the lower price range is an example of a simple app that can be used to teach children how to request and name items in their environment. It is easy to use and pictures familiar to the child can be added. Proloquo2go is an example of a more sophisticated app that can be used with older individuals or non-verbal students with well-developed literacy skills. It is important to remember though, that to use the more advanced, text-to-speech VOCAs, it is necessary to be able to type, spell, and have language in mind to communicate. Just giving a nonspeaking child a VOCA will not help him communicate unless he has these necessary skills. Many preverbal children with ASD will need to start with simpler systems, such as picture apps or physical boards with slots for pictures, in which they can point to one of a few pictures they would like to request. They might then move up to sets of cards they can line up to produce simple sentences, combining a picture representing "I want," for example, with a picture of their favorite snack or toy. VOCAs with pictorial options can be used for this purpose and may "speak" the picture's meaning. Research such as that done by Kasari's group (2014) suggests that this approach can assist with the development of language skills in children with ASD who are not yet speaking. Research on these approaches is in its infancy, but there is emerging evidence for them at this time, and they appear promising.

Sets of picture cards also can be used as a first step in order to help decide whether an electronic device would be worth the investment for the child. Many children with ASD love swiping on a tablet and watching how the visual display changes, but it is important to be sure that these activities are leading to functional growth in communication or other skills, rather than simply serving as an entertaining display. If the child seems to just enjoy the sensations of swiping and seeing, then this certainly can be used as a form of reinforcement for participating in more functional activities, but it is wise to be vigilant about whether the device is truly being used to enhance learning.

WHAT OTHER TREATMENTS ARE AVAILABLE BUT HAVE LESS ESTABLISHED EVIDENCE OF EFFICACY?

As we've seen, there are quite a number of techniques that have a reasonable degree of evidence for treating symptoms of ASD. Nonetheless, there are many, many more approaches that you will hear about from other families or on the Internet that may sound useful. While no evidence of efficacy is not, of course, the same as evidence of no efficacy, it is still important to be aware of which approaches have a stronger scientific base. We will mention here just a few of the methods for treating ASD that you are likely to encounter that cannot yet claim this basis in evidence.

Sensory-Motor Approaches

Sensory Integration   Many children with ASD are over- or undersensitive to sensations; some children are oversensitive to some stimuli and undersensitive to others. Parents often notice that their child with ASD doesn't respond when people speak to him or her and may fear the child is deaf, whereas other children (or sometimes the same child) can be overly upset by certain noises that don't seem to bother anyone else. Children with ASD may seem to avoid looking at people's faces but be captivated by small objects others hardly notice, or they may seem to dislike being touched but love to rub their fingers on certain textures or surfaces. Many variations of these sensory oddities can occur for any of the senses. Many children with ASD show odd motor patterns, too, such as enjoying spinning around, walking on tiptoes, flapping their hands, or using unusual postures. Some also have difficulties with oral-motor skills and have trouble learning to drink from a straw or cup or show unusual reactions to certain food textures. Unfortunately, not much is known about why these abnormalities tend to occur in ASD or what they mean for the child's prognosis or learning.

Some forms of treatment for ASD employ sensory diets, massaging, brushing, swinging, or other attempts to normalize or work around sensorimotor issues. Some make use of sensory rooms with ball pits, colored lights, music, and varied surfaces to explore. The weighted vests previously mentioned are another example of this approach. Although some children may enjoy the stimulation provided by these activities, and it's true that swinging or a massage may temporarily calm a child who is anxious or upset, there is no evidence that the effect carries over to enhance learning or reduce sensorimotor abnormalities for any period of time. If a child is upset, then it certainly makes sense to do something calming. If swinging calms a child, then there is no harm in it. If your child enjoys brushing or massaging, then by all means use it to create a pleasant, positive interaction time. It's important to know, though, that no convincing evidence has been produced to substantiate the claim that providing a child with a sensory diet or special environment of any kind for a certain amount of time every day will have any long-term effects on learning or behavior.

Prompts for Restructuring Oral Muscular Phonetic Targets   Prompts for Restructuring Oral Muscular Phonetic Targets (PROMPT) is a sensorimotor-based approach to developing speech skills for people with minimal or disordered speech production. It originally was developed to work with adults who lost speech ability as a result of a stroke. The originators later expanded its use to children with unintelligible speech as well as those with ASD. The idea behind PROMPT is to retrain neuromotor pathways, originally those that were damaged by stroke, through the use of tactile-kinesthetic cues provided by a therapist touching a child's face and neck. Although PROMPT has been in use since the 1980s, there is relatively little evidence published regarding its efficacy, and only one study has been done with children with ASD. This study showed little difference in outcome between children who received PROMPT and those who received the same amount of naturalistic behavior therapy; and neither group showed dramatic increases in speech production. PROMPT may be an approach worthy of a trial for children with ASD who are not talking, but it is by no means a guarantee that speech will be acquired. Other methods can work equally well as long as they are structured and intensive.

CAN PARENTS DELIVER TREATMENT OR ARE PROFESSIONALS BETTER?

Parents of young children are often involved in delivering intervention because young children often spend more time with parents than they do in a school or therapy setting, and parents may provide more consistent, intensive doses of therapy. Yet, many of the treatments discussed require some training and practice before they can be effectively delivered. Parents also usually have a lot of other things they need to do besides therapy, such as providing care and food for the child, taking care of other children, managing a household, and holding down a job. The combination of limited training and experience with multiple conflicting demands on their time makes it hard for many parents to consistently put in the intensive therapy time a child needs.

What does the scientific evidence say about the effectiveness of parents as opposed to trained therapists?

The answers aren't exactly clear. Studies looking at parents' ability to develop language skills in young children without autism generally support the effectiveness of parent-delivered intervention, but studies of parent-administered therapy for children with ASD tend to be less positive. One study from England found small effects of parental intervention over typical community treatment (Green et al., 2010); a study in the United States found parents improved their responsiveness to children after being trained to deliver therapy, but only the children who were lowest in terms of communication skills to start with showed improvements. Another study looked at parents' ability to deliver intervention on just one specific behavior—joint attention—and did find meaningful increases in the children's ability to engage in joint attention (Schertz & Odom, 2007). Many studies looking at the effects of early intervention in ASD combine direct therapist-delivered intervention with the training of parents to carry over the techniques beyond the therapist's direct service time. All these studies were conducted on children in the toddler age range, when parental involvement is thought to be most important. Not much is known about how parent-delivered therapy works for other age ranges. Public policy for children with ASD usually provides school-based programs for children once they turn 3 years old, so programs of intervention primarily delivered by parents typically are focused on children who are younger than 3 years old. Many birth-to-3 providers devote a significant amount of their service time to training parents to work with their children.

Is this practice justified by evidence? Would the time be better spent providing direct service to children, even if those services were limited to the hours therapists can be in the child's home?

Again, the answers are not clear-cut. Current, limited scientific evidence seems to suggest is that some degree of direct therapist involvement is useful in comprehensive intervention programs, even for very young children. Parents have difficulty being the primary intervention agents when a broad range of skills are being targeted. Parents seem more effective when trained to teach a specific skill, such as joint attention or imitation, with specific techniques and strategies, but other interventions also will be necessary in this case because children with ASD have a need for a broad range of educational treatments. It is also likely that comprehensive programs that include a parent training component will be more effective than those that do not because even preschool and school-age children with ASD will need parents to support the school program at home in more direct and intensive ways than are necessary for typically developing children. Including parent training that focuses on a small set of specific skills within a broader educational program is likely to be useful.

Bottom line: Once your young child is diagnosed with ASD, the intervention program should include evidence-based educational practices that target the range of skills previously mentioned as being central to improving social-communication in ASD (e.g., imitation, joint attention, play, gaze management, listening to speech, nonverbal and verbal communication). Trained professional therapists should be engaged in planning the program, based on their assessment findings, and delivering a portion of the service. In addition, the professionals should provide family members with some training in working with the child on a few specific targets. They should not only show the parent what to do, but should also work alongside parents, modeling strategies and taking turns so parents can try to make use of the model, giving feedback and encouraging questions and elaboration. They'll need to stay involved and oversee progress by observing either live or recorded samples of the parent working with the child and providing additional feedback, suggestions, and discussion. They also will need to monitor the child's progress in achieving each of the goals of the therapy. A mix of therapist-delivered intervention with parent-administered practice on a few skills that is overseen by a professional is the best suggestion based on our currently limited knowledge of best practices in treating young children with ASD.

You may be wondering how you are going to find time to give therapy to your child and still make time for your other children, your job, and your household chores. The good news is that you don't always have to set aside special time for working with your child. Many of your daily routines can serve as settings for practicing your child's target skills. You can ask your therapists for suggestions on how to conduct the activities they suggest in the context of everyday routines. For example, if you are working with your child on imitation, then bath time is a fun opportunity for encouraging mimicking washing hands, pushing a rubber duck, using a washcloth on knees, and lathering shampoo (it's also a great chance to emphasize the words for each of these actions to help develop your child's understanding of vocabulary). You can use hand-over-hand prompts at first and praise any attempts to imitate. If you are working on joint attention, then your child can help you pair up socks when they come out of the dryer. You can lay out all the socks, pick one up, then look at, point to, and direct your child's attention to its buddy and get him or her to hand it to you. You can gradually reduce the cues you use to direct attention until the child can follow just your gaze cue to find the buddy. You eventually can have the child pick a sock and direct your attention to its buddy. Other daily routines, such as picking what clothes to wear, choosing what toys to play with, or choosing utensils to help set the table can be done the same way. Once you begin, you will find yourself discovering a lot of opportunities to incorporate your child's developing social-communication skills into daily routines because these skills are used all the time in all normal interactions (that's why your child needs to learn them). If you find yourself with a few free moments, then you can play with your child, being mindful of the social-communication skills you want him or her to learn. Common infant games, such as Peekaboo, So big, and Pat-a-cake, and songs, such as "The Itsy-Bitsy Spider" and "Wheels on the Bus," are perfect for practicing looking at each other, imitating, taking turns, making sounds together, and saying first words.

These activities are still appropriate for toddlers and preschoolers with ASD who may not have been able to participate in them when they were younger. Playing with toys is also a great practice setting; and if you have other children, then they can be just as good a teacher as you once you show them some simple ways to help their sibling with ASD. You or your other children can have your child with ASD choose a toy (e.g., a car), demonstrate how to use it, encourage imitation of the right way to use the toy for a few turns (e.g., imitate rolling a car instead of turning it upside down), then allow a short turn for the child with ASD to use the toy in the preferred way before going back to imitating you or a sibling. Although you may need to supervise this play at first, you are likely to find that your other children come to enjoy being a teacher for their sibling and will take as much pride in new accomplishments as you do. You can talk with your therapist about ways you and your other children can use play settings to practice the skills you are targeting.

HOW MANY HOURS OF TREATMENT DOES YOUR CHILD NEED?

There was a time when claims were made that only 40 hours of intervention was adequate, regardless of the child's age. Research has shown, however, that 20 hours of intervention is just as effective as 40 hours for young children; there is only so much a young child can absorb. Still, there are few hard-and-fast rules about how much intervention is enough at what age. School-age children typically will receive the standard 30 or so hours per week that make up a typical school schedule. The National Research Council (2001) recommended 15–25 hours per week for young children, but it also depends on your child. For 3- to 5-year-olds, 15–25 hours a week is reasonable, but many will have to work up to it, starting out with half days or 2–3 days a week in school and gradually adjusting to a more intensive schedule. Young 3-year-olds may still need a nap in the afternoon and may not be able to participate in a full-day program. Few children younger than 3 years old will receive this level of programming, and some could not tolerate it even if it were available. A child who is younger than 3 years old should see a professional therapist at least 4–5 days per week, for 1–2 hours per day, depending on the child's tolerance, and following up with some focused parent–child interaction working on therapy goals for at least 30 minutes almost every day.

Therapists in birth-to-3 programs often cross-treat, meaning that they consult with each other and teach each other how to implement each other's strategies. For example, the OT and SLP might work together to develop a plan to help your child learn to tolerate more food textures. The OT might see your child twice a week to work on fine motor skills, as well as feeding, using the strategies planned with the SLP. The SLP might visit the child twice a week and work on feeding, using the same strategies, along with gestures and vocal communication. Your child would be seeing professional therapists four times per week, and their services would overlap, even though the child would be seeing each therapist only twice a week. Both therapists would work with parents to help them implement the feeding strategies throughout the week at mealtimes so that feeding skills could be practiced when the therapists weren't present. This level of programming is appropriate for most toddlers with ASD.

Apart from the total number of hours of intervention a child receives, parents often worry about how much of each type of intervention the child gets. For example, if the SLP is only seeing the child once a week, then parents may feel the child is not getting enough communication intervention. This may be true, but it is not necessarily so. What really matters is not how many hours a particular therapist spends with your child, but the more important questions to consider are

- What does the therapist do while with your child?

- Are the goals functional and easily related to real-world activities?

- Are the methods evidence based?

- Is progress regularly tracked so changes can be made if the program isn't working and new goals targeted as the child progresses?

- Can the therapist manage your child's behavior so that most of the time is spent on practicing skills and not dealing with misbehavior?

- Does the therapist provide the family with a small, doable set of activities to carry over therapy activities at home, with periodic progress reports (outside of formal meetings) and opportunities to discuss questions and concerns?

- Does the therapist work closely with the rest of the child's team so everyone knows what targets and techniques are being used and do all team members exchange ideas about how to address goals as they work on their own? If the child is in school, does the therapist work closely with the classroom teacher so the teacher provides opportunities for your child to work on targets within the classroom setting? Does the therapist suggest ways for your child to work or play with other children so that target skills are practiced?

It may not be necessary for a particular therapist to see your child every day if the therapist's activities are structured so that for your child can practice important skills with you or other therapists. Many therapists have the skills needed to address the basic social-communication development that is most important for a child with ASD, especially a young child. Just because your child may not see the SLP each day does not mean communication skills won't be addressed. The PT might consult with the SLP and emphasize words for body parts during sessions with your child, perhaps playing "Head, Shoulders, Knees, and Toes" to emphasize vocabulary and increase body awareness and flexibility. The OT could consult with the SLP and work on color words as your child learns to hold crayons appropriately during drawing activities. The ABA therapist may choose object names to teach based on the SLP's recommendations while using DTI drills. If these kinds of collaborations are going on, then it may not be crucial for the SLP to have a daily session with your child. If they aren't, then it may be more important to advocate for more collaboration among your team than for more hours from one particular therapist.

FIRST, DO NO HARM

We've talked a lot about the importance of scientific evidence in choosing interventions for your child with ASD. Many treatments are available that have little or no scientific evidence because ASD is such a serious disorder and it is relatively widespread. There are also many purported cures for other serious, common diseases, such as cancer, and information about them has become even more accessible with the Internet. But think about it. If apricot pits, herbal medicine, or shark cartilage were really helpful in treating cancer, don't you think some doctor or company would have found a way to treat people and make them better and wouldn't reputable sources have followed up on the claims and made them public knowledge? Is it reasonable to believe there is a cure for a devastating disease that is being kept secret and not being investigated? It is highly unlikely. ASD cures fall into the same category. You will find many of them if you search the Internet: dolphin therapy, bee sting therapy, auditory integration therapy, hyperbaric chambers, gluten-free/casein-free diets, megavitamin therapy, prism glasses, parasitic worms, hippotherapy, treatment for leaky gut syndrome, and chelation. Some of these have been subjected to scientific study and found to be useless; that hasn't stopped their proliferation on the Internet. It also won't stop other parents from urging you to try things like this that they feel have worked or are working for their child. Of course you don't want to miss the chance that some of these unlikely cures will help. You may ask yourself, "What have we got to lose?"

Not Much to Lose

You're right. There may be little to lose in trying an alternative therapy if it will set your mind at ease. Therapies that manipulate diet may not do much harm, but be sure to carefully monitor the effects. First, check with your child's doctor and explain the diet in detail so the doctor can be sure it won't harm the child or impede physical growth or development. Start slowly, eliminating one food at a time, so you can see what, if anything, makes a difference. Keep written records; it is easy to forget how a child behaved last week or 6 weeks ago. Remember that symptoms naturally wax and wane; it is easy to attribute a change to your intervention when it might just be part of the natural course of the condition.

To get your best shot at learning whether the treatment makes a difference, ask teachers or therapists to give you a brief report of how your child is doing before starting the alternative treatment and again a couple of weeks after making the changes. After the child has been on the complete regimen for a month or 6 weeks, withdraw the treatment and ask your raters to give you another report to see whether things get worse. If at all possible, don't tell your observers when the child was on or off the treatment. Remember discussing the importance of blind raters? If people know the child is trying a new treatment, then they will be more likely to think they see changes. Try to get information from people who aren't aware what treatment the child is or is not getting. Using a method like this will allow you to get a fairly clear picture of whether the treatment makes a real difference. It is always worthwhile to make an effort to find out if what you are doing works. You wouldn't want to subject a child to it unless it has real value.

Vitamins can be expensive, there is a potential for overdosing, and your child may not like taking them. Try them only with your doctor's collaboration and monitor their effects. The same is true for medications your doctor may prescribe to control symptoms of ASD. You need to know whether a prescription medication is working as planned just as much as you do a diet or supplement. Try to get blind raters to let you know if they see changes when the child is on versus off the medication. After discussing your plan with your doctor, don't be afraid to stop the medication for a week, once the child has taken it for a month, and see whether things go downhill. All medicines have some side effects and you don't want to expose your child to them unless there is a clear benefit to taking the medication. Mainstream medicines should be evaluated as carefully as an alternative approach.

Riskier Business

Some of the alternative therapies you will read about are at a somewhat higher level of risk. In most cases, the risk is to your finances. Dolphin therapy costs more than $2,000 for 5 days of participation, and although your child with ASD, like your other children, may enjoy swimming with dolphins, there is absolutely no evidence of any long-term effects of the experience. Auditory integration therapy, which involves having children listen through headphones to specially filtered music for two 30-minute sessions a day for 10 days also has no evidence of behavioral effects and is very costly. Prism glasses and other forms of vision therapy are prescribed by eye doctors. Although some parents swear by them, there is no scientific evidence that they do any good. Try them if you want, but carefully monitor their effects and don't spend a lot of money on them. Hippotherapy, or therapeutic horseback riding, is another alternative therapy in which there is not much to lose. It is usually inexpensive, can be enjoyable for many children with and without ASD, and may provide some improvements in balance and posture. Again, there is no evidence that it has any effect on the core symptoms of ASD.

Some of the purported therapies for ASD rest on the idea that autism is an immune disorder and the immune system needs to be stimulated. Bee sting therapy, parasitic worm therapy, hyperbaric therapy, and therapies for leaky gut syndrome aim to address this need. Although it is true that some studies have shown immune abnormalities in some (not all) children with ASD, it is not clear if or how these abnormalities contribute to the behaviors associated with the disorder, so it's hard to know how stimulating the immune system would help. There also are no convincing reports of improvement in particular ASD symptoms following their use. It seems risky to disturb a biological system so central to overall health when it isn't clear there is a problem. Given the uncertainties of biological and behavioral effects of immune-based therapies, the risk seems to outweigh their very questionable benefit.

Dangerous Territory

Some alternative therapies can involve serious dangers. Chelation, the attempt to remove heavy metals claimed to be toxic to the brain from the bloodstream, has resulted in the deaths of several children with ASD.

Facilitated communication, an apparently harmless attempt to provide a channel of communication to individuals who are nonverbal by guiding them to point to letters on a letter board or type on a keyboard, has resulted in a host of bizarre accusations of abuse and sexual molestation allegedly produced by the person with ASD. These allegations resulted in the arrest of accused family members and removal of children from their families and placement in foster care. Later court proceedings demonstrated that it was the facilitator who was unconsciously producing the communication and that the accusations were fabricated by the facilitator, albeit unconsciously. Although facilitators sincerely believed their client with ASD was sending complex, literate messages through facilitation, controlled studies demonstrated clearly that when the facilitator was shown one object and the person with autism (covertly) shown a different one, invariably the person with ASD appeared to type the name of the object only the facilitator saw. This episode demonstrates the hidden dangers of even apparently innocent interventions and the crucial need to objectively establish that a particular intervention is valid, safe, and effective. Recent reports of a return to this method (http://blog.asha.org/2015/05/19/the-pseudoscientific-phenom-facilitated-communication-makes-a-comeback/) suggest caution about it is still warranted.

CONCLUSION

This chapter aimed to elaborate why it is so important to establish the effectiveness of whatever intervention your child is receiving, whether it be ABA, medication, speech, occupational or physical therapy, or alternative medicine. It reviewed what the scientific literature reports about some of the most well-known intervention approaches. Most of all, the chapter encouraged you to ensure that therapies used with your child are monitored and evaluated in order to make sure they are working to alleviate symptoms and enhance learning. A few take-away points have emerged from this discussion:

- Parents have the right to question their child's educational team about the evidence available for the methods they've chosen, using questions provided here to start discussions.

- Children with ASD can benefit from a range of therapeutic approaches; there is not one right way. Still, some approaches have more evidence behind them than others. These methods should be a part of every child's program. Less established interventions can be added when they closely match the child's needs and preferences, but they must be carefully monitored to ensure they are working.

- Parents can be effective agents of intervention, particularly for young children, but they are most likely to be successful when given focused training and feedback in using specific techniques to address specific targets and when they work closely with professionals to monitor progress.

- Children with ASD need structured, intensive interactions in order to learn, but there is no magic number of hours that guarantee success. Hours should gradually increase as the child approaches school age. Being sure that therapists work together to integrate the child's goals into a range of activities and that parents have clear guidance about carrying over the strategies in daily routines is more important than how many hours the child sees each team member.

- Parents have the right to try alternative therapies, even when the scientific evidence does not support them, but they should consult with the child's doctors, teachers, and therapists to make sure the therapies do no harm. They should monitor the effects of any therapy, ask people to rate the child when the raters don't know if the child is on or off the intervention protocol, and make every effort to evaluate whether the therapy is having a meaningful effect.

- Although providing the most effective intervention for the child with ASD is clearly important, the rest of the family is important, too. Families should not devote all their financial and emotional resources to the child with ASD, but they need to balance his or her needs with those of the rest of the family. The child with ASD does best in the long run when the family is strong and healthy. We take care of our children most effectively when we take care of ourselves as well.

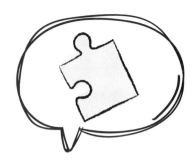

Epilogue

We hope that you are now feeling more equipped to face the challenges that come with having a child with autism in the family. We're certain, however, that you still have a lot of questions in your mind. Will your child go to kindergarten? Will your child graduate from high school? Go to college? Live independently as an adult? You may have no way of knowing the answers to all these questions yet, but many parents can't help thinking about them.

Let's take the easy question first: Will your child go to kindergarten? The answer to this is almost certainly yes. Public schools are legally obligated to provide free appropriate public education for all children, and many students with ASD participate in regular kindergarten programs with varying levels of support from special educators and therapists. Some parents prefer not to send their child to mainstream kindergarten but keep them in a special education setting because they believe their child will receive more intensive, individualized instruction. Most parents who want their child to have a chance to try inclusive education can get agreement at least at the kindergarten level. You will want to work with your school to decide whether your child can benefit from the mainstream curriculum in order to decide what kind of placement makes the most sense. The kindergarten experience can often help you make a rational decision. Even if your child doesn't spend the whole day in an inclusive setting, there will still be opportunities for interaction throughout the day to interact with typically developing peers.

When you think about the other questions, we encourage you to remember that you won't know the answer to all these questions about a typically developing child, either. For example, one of our children, a typically developing but academically uninterested teenager, left us on the eve of his high school commencement ceremony with no idea whether he would graduate. He appeared constitutionally (though in no way neurologically) unable to pass a math course or a math final throughout his high school career. It wasn't until the night before commencement that we learned he had managed to get a *D* on the final math exam (most likely as a result of charity, coupled with a desire never to have him in a class again, on the part of his teacher) and would indeed graduate with his class. Many of the concerns you feel are unique to having a child with ASD may not be as different as you think.

You also may be surprised at how much delight you will feel about what your child with ASD does accomplish. We know of families of adults with ASD who have told us how intensely proud they feel of their grown children who live in their own apartment or have a job helping out in the student union at the local college or copying documents at the library. These may not be the dreams you thought you would have for your child, but they may turn out to be great accomplishments that allow your child to experience self-sufficiency, contribute to the community, and enjoy a life that accommodates most needs and desires. These are the elements that make a life happy, and isn't that really what we all want for our children, a way to find happiness within their abilities?

Perhaps, underneath, this is really what you worry about—whether your child will find a way to grow up to be happy. Again, we never know this for any child, but we certainly hope it for all of them. Happiness may look different for someone with ASD than it does for others. It's true that some young people with ASD lament a lack of friends or romantic relationships, but some will be quite content to be allowed to pursue their own interests and relish their solitude. Some may welcome the freedom from social skills training and educational interventions aimed to help them be more like others and find satisfaction in just being themselves. We have met many adults with ASD whose lives may look limited from the outside but who find contentment, even within a somewhat narrow sphere.

We think of a young man with autism we know who works delivering mail from the mailroom to various departments at a local hospital. "Jay-Jay" has a script he goes through at each department where he delivers the mail; each day he says the same thing to each person and each time he says it, his smile is as broad as if he'd just won the lottery. Everyone looks forward to seeing him, and if he misses a day of work, everyone wants to know where he is and when he'll be back. Jay-Jay has lived in his own apartment, but after a while he decided he preferred to live at home with his parents. With their other children grown and flown, they enjoy having him as a roommate and appreciate his help with preparing meals and gardening.

We also know several intelligent people with ASD who live fulfilling lives that, even if they don't include a lot of friends or marriage, include meaningful work, social interactions around shared interests, and in some cases a certain degree of fame related to their unusual accomplishments. Temple Grandin, subject of an HBO biopic, and Daniel Tammet, who holds the European record for reciting pi from memory to 22,514 digits in 5 hours, come to mind.

Even if your child does not grow up to be famous, though, you should re-member that the opportunities for people with ASD are much more varied and open today than they ever have been, thanks to the efforts and courage of fami-lies who have raised money for research, lobbied for legislative changes, banded together for mutual support, and bravely shrugged when their child acted out and just explained that the child had autism. It is the insistence of families that the rest of us understand and accept their children that has led to the enormous changes that have happened in the recent past and will continue to expand op-portunities for people who don't fit the common mold.

What if you find you cannot manage your child or adult with ASD at home, despite all of your efforts? We know many families feel this would be a tragic outcome, but again, try to remember that happiness for your child with ASD may not look the same as happiness for others. We know of at least one family of a boy with ASD who struggled for years to keep him at home and found that it became impossible when he was entering puberty. At first they were wracked with guilt and shame, but they were able to place him in a residential program where he thrived, to their astonishment. An environment governed by rules that provides complete consistency, predictability, and safety in the way a fam-ily home cannot is the most comfortable environment and one in which some people with severe autism may feel for the first time that the world behaves in a way that makes sense. Just as some families of typically developing children feel a residential school provides certain advantages, at some point your family may feel this way too. If that time ever comes, then you will not have failed; instead, you will have become willing to make the difficult sacrifice of permitting your child to live away from home in order to reap the benefits of a setting that pro-vides for his or her needs.

There is no denying the fact that being the parents of a child with ASD takes courage, determination, a lot of time, and energy. It's not a job anyone signs up for, but it can be one that brings its own kind of fulfillment. Our hope is that you will find this fulfillment for your family when you are armed with informa-tion and understanding about ASD.

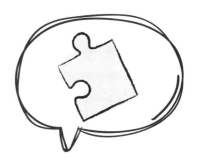

References

Akbar, M., Loomis, R., & Paul, R. (2013). The interplay of language and executive functions in children with ASD. *Research in Autism Spectrum Disorders, 7,* 494–501.

American Psychiatric Association (1968). *Diagnostic and statistical manual of mental diseases* (2nd ed.). Washington, DC: Author.

American Psychiatric Association (1994). *Diagnostic and statistical manual of mental diseases* (4th ed.). Washington, DC: Author.

American Psychiatric Association. (2013). *Diagnostic and statistical manual of mental disorders* (5th ed.). Washington DC: Author.

Arick, J., Young, H., Falco, R., Loos, L., Krug, D., Gense, M., & Johnson, S. (2003). Designing an outcome study to monitor the progress of students with autism spectrum disorders. *Focus on Autism and Other Developmental Disabilities, 18,* 75–87.

Asperger, H. (1944/1991). Die "autistischen Psyopathen" im Kindesalter. *Archives fur Psychiatrie und Nervenkrankheiten, 117,* 76–136. Translated by Frith, U. (Ed.). (1991). *Autism and Asperger's syndrome.* Cambridge, UK: University Press.

Bauminger-Zviely, N. (2014). School-age children with ASD. In F. Volkmar, S. Rogers, R. Paul, & K. Pelphrey (Eds.), *Handbook of autism and PDD* (4th ed.; pp. 148–175). New York, NY: Wiley.

Bayley, N. (2005). *Bayley Scales of Infant and Toddler Development, Third Edition (BSID-III).* San Antonio, TX: Pearson/PsychCorp.

Beilinson, J., & Olswang, L. (2003). Facilitating peer-group entry in kindergartners with impairments in social communication. *Language, Speech, and Hearing Services in Schools, 34*(2), 157.

Berbert, M. (Producer), & Truffaut, F. (Director). (1970). *L'Enfant sauvage.* France: Les Films du Carrosse.

Bleiweiss, J., Hough, L., & Cohen, S. (2013). *Everyday classroom strategies and practices for supporting children with autism spectrum disorders.* Shawnee Mission, KS: Autism Asperger Publishing Company.

Bloom, L. (1993). *The transition from infancy to language: Acquiring the power of expression.* Cambridge, UK: Cambridge University Press.

Boersma, M., Kemner, C., de Reus, M.A., Collin, G., Snijders, T.M., Hofman, D., & van den Heuvel, M.P. (2012). Disrupted functional brain networks in autistic toddlers. *Brain Connectivity, 3*(1), 41–49. doi:10.1089/brain.2012.0127

Bricker, D., Capt, B., Johnson, J., Pretti-Frontczak, K., Waddell, M., & Straka, E. (2002). *Assessment, Evaluation, and Programming System for Infants and Children (AEPS®), Second Edition, 4-Volume Set.* Baltimore, MD: Paul H. Brookes Publishing Co.

Brigance, A. (2004). *Brigance Inventory of Early Development, Second Edition (IED-II).* North Billerica, MA: Curriculum Associates.

Briggs-Gowan, M., & Carter, A. (2006). *Brief Infant-Toddler Social and Emotional Assessment (BITSEA).* San Antonio, TX: PsychCorp.

Bryson, S., Zwaigenbaum, L., McDermott, C., Rombough, V., & Brian, J. (2008). The Autism Observation Scale for Infants: Scale development and reliability data. *Journal of Autism and Developmental Disorders, 38,* 731–738.

Bzoch, K., League, R., & Brown, V. (2003). *Receptive-Expressive Emergent Language Scale–Third Edition (REEL-3).* Austin, TX: PRO-ED.

Campbell, S., Cannon, B., Ellis, J.T., Lifter, K., Luiselli, J.K., Navalta, C.P., Tara, M. (1998). The May Center for early childhood education: Description of a continuum of services model for children with autism. *International Journal of Disability, Development and Education, 45,* 173–187.

Chapman, R. (2008). *The everyday guide to special education law: A handbook for parents, teachers and other professionals* (2nd ed.). Grand Junction, CO: The Legal Center for People with Disabilities and Older People.

Cohen, H., Amerine-Dickens, M., & Smith, T. (2006). Early intensive behavioral treatment: Replication of the UCLA model in a community setting. *Developmental and Behavioral Pediatrics, 27*(2), 145–155.

Cohen, M. (2009). *A guide to special education advocacy.* London, England: Jessica Kingsley Publishers.

Collins, A., & Dworkin, R. (2011). Pilot study of the effectiveness of weighted vests. *American Journal of Occupational Therapy, 65*(6), 688–694.

Cox, A., Gast, D., Juscre, D., & Ayres, K. (2009). The effects of weighted vests on appropriate in-seat behaviors of elementary-age students with autism and severe to profound intellectual disabilities. *Focus on Autism and Other Developmental Disabilities, 24*(1), 17–26.

Danovich, J., Paul, R., Volkmar, F. & Klin, A. (April, 2009). *Developmental trajectories of special interests in children with ASD.* Denver, CO: Society for Research in Child Development.

Dawson, G., Rogers, S., Munson, J., Smith, M., Winter, J., Greenson, J. . . . Varley, J. (2010). Randomized, controlled trial of an intervention for toddlers with autism: The Early Start Denver model. *Pediatrics, 125*(1), 17–23.

De Giacomo, A, & Fombonne, E. (1998). Parental recognition of developmental abnormalities in autism. *European Child and Adolescent Psychiatry, 7*(3), 131–136.

Dietz, C., Swinkel, S., van Daalen, E., van Engeland, H., & Buitelaar, J. (2006). Screening for autism spectrum disorder in children aged 14–15 months II: Population screening with the Early Screening for Autistic Traits Questionnaire (ESAT) design and general findings. *Journal of Autism and Developmental Disorders, 36,* 713–722.

Dunlap, G., Iovannone, R., English, C., Kincaid, D., Wilson, K., Christiansen, K., & Strain, P. (2010). *Prevent-teach-reinforce: A school-based model of individualized positive behavior support.* Baltimore, MD: Paul H. Brookes Publishing Co.

Dunn, L., and Dunn, L. (2006). *Peabody Picture Vocabulary Test—IV.* Circle Pines, MN: American Guidance Service.

Eaves, L., & Ho, H. (2004). The very early identification of autism: Outcome to age $4\frac{1}{2}$–5. *Journal of Autism and Developmental Disorders, 34,* 367–378.

Edwards, S., Fletcher, P., Garman, M., Hughes, A., Letts, C., & Sinka, I. (1999). *Reynell Developmental Language Scales III.* Windsor, United Kingdom: NFER-Nelson.

English, K., Shafer, K., Goldstein, H., & Kaczmarek, L. (1997). Teaching buddy skills to preschoolers. *Innovations: American Association on Mental Retardation, research to practice series.*

Fahim, D. (2011, November). *Toddlers with autism spectrum disorders: A workshop on intervention strategies and best practices for families and providers.* Washington DC: National Drug Endangered Children Conference.

Fein, D., Barton, M., Eigsti, I., Kelley, E., Naigles, L., Schultz, R. . . . Tyson, K. (2013). Optimal outcome in individuals with a history of autism. *Journal of Child Psychology and Psychiatry, 54,* 195–205.

Fenske, E.C., Zalenski, S., Krantz, P.J., & McClannahan, L.E. (1985). Age at intervention and treatment outcome for autistic children in a comprehensive intervention program. *Analysis and Intervention in Developmental Disabilities, 5,* 49–58.

Fenson, L., Marchman, V.A., Thal, D.J., Dale, P.S., Reznick, S., & Bates, E. (2006). *The MacArthur-Bates Communicative Development Inventories user's guide and technical manual, second edition.* Baltimore, MD: Paul H. Brookes Publishing Co.

Ferguson, F., Saines, E. (Producers), & Jackson, M. (Director). (2010). *Temple Grandin.* USA: HBO Films.

Fey, M., Justice, L. & Schmitt, M. (2014). Evidence-based decision making in communication intervention. In R. Paul (Ed.) *Introduction to clinical methods in communication disorders*. Baltimore, MD: Paul H. Brookes Publishing Co.

Freeman, S., & Dake, L. (1996). *Teach me language: A language manual for children with autism, Asperger's syndrome and related disorders*. Bellingham, WA: SKF Books.

Gilliam, J. (2006). *Gilliam Autism Rating Scales, Second Edition*. Los Angeles, CA: Western Psychological Services.

Glover, M., Preminger, J., & Sanford, A. (2002). *Early Learning Accomplishment Profile (Early-LAP/ELAP)*. Lewisville, NC: Kaplan Early Learning.

Grandin, T. (2006). *Thinking in pictures: My life with autism*. New York, NY: Vintage Books.

Gray, C. (1994). *Comic book conversations*. Arlington, TX: Future Horizons.

Gray, C., & Attwood, T. (2010). *The new social story book–revised and expanded*. Arlington, TX: Future Horizons.

Green, J., Charman, T., McConachie, H., Aldred, C., Slonims, V., Howlin, P., Le Couteur, A. . . . Pickles, A. (2010). Parent-mediated communication-focused treatment in children with autism (PACT): A randomised controlled trial. *The Lancet, 375*(9732), 2152–2160.

Greenspan, S., & Wieder, S. (1998). *The child with special needs: Encouraging intellectual and emotional growth*. Boston, MA: Da Capo Press

Greenspan, S., & Weider, S. (2006). *Engaging autism*. Philadelphia, PA: Perseus Books.

Gutstein, S.E., Burgess, A.F., & Montfort, K. (2007). Evaluation of the relationship development intervention. *Autism, 11*, 397–411.

Gutstein, S. & Sheely, R., (2002). *Relationship Development Intervention with Young Children: Social and Emotional Development Activities for Asperger Syndrome, Autism, PDD and NLD*. Philadelphia, PA: Jessica Kingsley Publishers.

Hancock, T., and Kaiser, A. (2006). Enhanced milieu teaching. In McCauley, R. & Fey, M. (Eds.), *Treatment of language disorders in children* (pp. 203–236). Baltimore, MD: Paul H. Brookes Publishing Co.

Happe, R., & Firth, U. (2006). The weak coherence account: Detail-focused cognitive style in autism spectrum disorders. *Journal of Autism and Developmental Disorders, 36*, 5–25.

Harris, S.L., & Handleman, J.S. (2000). Age and IQ at intake as predictors of placement for young children with autism: A four- to six-year follow-up. *Journal of Autism and Developmental Disorders, 30*(2), 137–142.

Health Care and Education Reconciliation Act of 2010, P.L. 111-152. 124, Stat. 1029.

Hedrick, D., Prather, E., & Tobin, A. (1995). *Sequenced Inventory of Communication Development—Revised (SICD-R)*. Los Angeles, CA: Western Psychological Services.

Heumer, S., & Mann, V. (2010). A comprehensive profile of decoding and comprehension in autism spectrum disorders. *Journal of Autism and Developmental Disorders, 40* 485–493

Hill, A., Zuckerman, K., & Fombonne, E. (2014). Epidemiology of autism spectrum disorders. In F. Volkmar, S. Rogers, R. Paul, & K. Pelphrey (Eds.), *Handbook of autism and pervasive developmental disorders* (4th ed.; pp. 57–96). New York, NY: Wiley.

Hodgetts, S., Magill-Evans, J., & Misiaszek, J. (2011). Weighted vests, stereotyped behaviors and arousal in children with autism. *Journal of Autism and Developmental Disorders, 41*(6), 805–814.

Howlin, P., Moss, P., Savage, S., & Rutter, M. (2013). Social outcomes in mid- to later adulthood among individuals diagnosed with autism and average nonverbal IQ as children. *Journal of the American Academy of Child and Adolescent Psychiatry, 52*(6), 572–581. doi:10.1016/j.jaac.2013.02.017

Hoyson, M., Jamieson, B., & Strain, P.S. (1984). Individualized group instruction of normally developing and autistic-like children: The LEAP curriculum model. *Journal of the Division for Early Childhood, 8*, 157–172.

Hresko, W., Reid, K., & Hammill, D. (1999). *Test of Early Language Development—Third Edition (TELD-3)*. San Antonio, TX: Pearson/Harcourt Assessment.

Hume, K.A., & Odom, S.L. (2011). Best practices, policy, and future directions: Behavioral and psychosocial interventions. In D. Amaral, G. Dawson, & D. Geschwind (Eds.), *Autism spectrum disorders* (pp. 1295–1308). New York, NY: Oxford University Press.

Ibrahim, S., Voight, R., Katusic, S., Weaver, A., & Barbaresi, W. (2009). Incidence of gastrointestinal symptoms in children with autism: A population-based study. *Pediatrics, 124*, 680–686.

Individuals with Disabilities Education Improvement Act (IDEA) of 2004, PL 108-446, 20 U.S.C. §§ 1400 *et seq*.

Jones, W., & Klin, A. (2013). Attention to eyes is present but in decline in 2- to 6-month-old infants later diagnosed with autism. *Nature, 504*(7480), 427–431. doi:10.1038/nature12715

Jusczyk, P. (2002). Some critical developments in acquiring native language sound organization during the first year. *Annals of Otology, Rhinology, and Laryngology Supplement, 189,* 11–25.

Kanner, L. (1943). Autistic disturbances of affective contact. *Nervous Child, 2,* 217–250.

Kasari, C., Gulsrud, A., Freeman, S., Paparella, T., & Hellemann, G. (2012). Longitudinal follow-up of children with autism receiving targeted interventions on joint attention and play. *Journal of the American Academy of Child and Adolescent Psychiatry, 51*(5), 487–495. doi:10.1016/j.jaac.2012.02.019

Kasari, C., Gulsrud, A.C., Wong, C., Kwon, S., & Locke, J. (2010). Randomized controlled caregiver mediated joint engagement intervention for toddlers with autism. *Journal of Autism and Developmental Disorders, 40,* 1045–1056.

Kasari, C., Kaiser, A., Goods, K. Nietfeld, J., Mathy, PP., Landa, R., Murphy, S. & Almirall, D. (2014). Communication interventions for minimally verbal children with autism: A sequential multiple assignment randomized trial. *Journal of the American Academy of Child and Adolescent Psychiatry, 53,* 635–646.

Kasari, C., Paparella, T., Freeman, S., & Jahromi, L. (2008). Language outcome in autism: Randomized comparison of joint attention and play interventions. *Journal of Consulting and Clinical Psychology, 76(1),* 125–137.

Keen, D., Couzens, D., Muspratt, S., & Rodger, S. (2010). The effects of a parent-focused intervention for children with a recent diagnosis of autism spectrum disorder on parenting stress and competence. *Research in Autism Spectrum Disorders, 4*(2), 229–241.

Kelley, E., Paul, J., Fein, D., & Naigles, L. (2006). Residual language deficits in optimal outcome children with a history of autism. *Journal of Autism and Developmental Disorders, 36,* 807–828.

Kleinman, J., Robins, D., Ventola, P., Pandey, J., Boorstein, H., Esser, E. . . . Fein, D. (2008). The modified checklist for autism in toddlers: A follow-up study investigating the early detection of autism spectrum disorders. *Journal of Autism and Developmental Disorders, 38,* 827–839.

Knott, F., Lewis, C. & Williams, T. (2007). Sibling interaction of children with autism: Development over 12 months. *Journal of Autism and Developmental Disorders, 37,* 1987–1995.

Koegel, R., & Koegel, L. (2006). *Pivotal Response Treatments for autism.* Baltimore, MD: Paul H. Brookes Publishing Co.

Koegel, L., Koegel, R., Miller, A., & Detar, W. (2014). Issues and interventions for ASD during adolescence and beyond. In F. Volkmar, S. Rogers, R. Paul, & K. Pelphrey (Eds.), *Handbook of autism and PDD* (4th ed.; pp. 176–190). New York, NY: Wiley.

Koenig, K., & Volkmar, F. (2012). *Practical social skills for autism spectrum disorders: Designing child-specific interventions.* New York, NY: W.W. Norton.

Landa, R. (2012). *Early signs of autism.* http://www.kennedykrieger.org/patient-care/patient-care-centers/center-autism-and-related-disorders/outreach-training/early-signs-of-autism-video-tutorial

Lane, H. (1979). *The wild boy of Averyron.* Cambridge, MA: Harvard University Press.

Lawton, K., & Kasari, C. (2012). Teacher-implemented joint attention intervention: Pilot randomized controlled study for preschoolers with autism. *Journal of Consulting and Clinical Psychology, 80,* 687–693.

Leew, S., Stein, N., & Gibbard, W. (2010). Weighted vests' effect on social attention for toddlers with Autism Spectrum Disorders. *Canadian Journal of Occupational Therapy, 77,* 113–124.

Linder, T.W. (2008). *Transdisciplinary Play-Based Assessment, Second Edition (TPBA2).* Baltimore, MD: Paul H. Brookes Publishing Co.

Lord, C., & McGee, J.P. (Eds.). (2001). *Educating children with autism.* Washington, DC: National Research Council.

Lord, C., Rutter, M., DiLavore, P., Risi, S., Gotham, K., & Bishop, S. (2012). *Autism Diagnostic Observation Scale* (2nd ed.). Los Angeles, CA: Western Psychological Services.

Lord, C., Shulman, C., & DiLavore, P. (2004). Regression and word loss in autistic spectrum disorders. *Journal of Child Psychology and Psychiatry, 45*(5), 936–955. doi:10.1111/j.1469-7610.2004.t01-1-00287.x

Lovaas, I. (1981). *The ME book.* Los Angeles, CA: The Lovaas Institute.

Lovaas, I. (1987). Behavioral treatment and normal educational and intellectual functioning in young autistic children. *Journal of Consulting and Clinical Psychology, 55,* 3–9.

Lucker, J. (2013). Auditory hypersensitivity in children with autism spectrum disorders. *Focus Autism Other Developmental Disabilities, 28*(3), 184–191.

Macintosh, K., & Dissanayake, C. (2006). A comparative study of the spontaneous social interactions of children with high functioning autism and children with Asperger's disorder. *Autism, 10,* 199–220.

Magiati, I., Wei, X., & Howlin, P. (2012). Early comprehensive behaviorally based interventions for children with autism spectrum disorders: a summary of findings from recent reviews and meta-analyses. *Neuropsychiatry, 6,* 543–570.

Magill-Evans, J., & Misiaszek, J. (2011). Weighted vests, stereotyped behaviors and arousal in children with autism. *Journal of Autism and Developmental Disorders, 41,* 805–814.

Mahoney, G., & Perales, F. (2005). Relationship-focused early intervention with children with pervasive developmental disorders and other disabilities: A comparative study. *Journal of Developmental and Behavioral Pediatrics, 26*(2), 77–85.

McClannahan, L., & Krantz, P. (2005). *Teaching conversation to children with autism: Scripts and script fading.* Bethesda, MD: Woodbine House.

McElhanin, B., McCracken, C., Karpen, S., & Shar, W. (2014). Gastrointestinal symptoms in autism spectrum disorder: A meta-analysis. *Pediatrics, 133,* 872–883.

Mesibov, G.B. (1997). Formal and informal measures on the effectiveness of the TEACCH programme. *Autism, 1*(1), 25–35.

Mesibov, G., Shea, V., Schopler, E., Adams, L., Merkler, E., Burgess, S. . . . Bourgondien, M. (2004). *The TEACCH approach to autism spectrum disorders.* New York, NY: Springer.

Mullen, E. (1995). *Mullen Scales of Early Learning (MSEL).* San Antonio, TX: Pearson.

Mundy, P., Delgado, C., Block, J., Venezia, M., Hogan, A., & Seibert, J. (2003). *Early social communication scales.* Miami, FL: University of Miami.

Munro, N., Lee, K., and Baker, E. (2008). Building vocabulary knowledge and phonological awareness skills in children with specific language impairment through hybrid language intervention: a feasibility study. *International Journal of Language and Communication Disorders, 43*(6), 662–682.

Nation, K., Clarke, Pl., Wright, B., & Williams, C. (2006). Patterns of reading ability in children with autism spectrum disorders *Journal of Autism and Developmental Disorders, 15,* 911–919.

National Research Council. (2001). *Educating children with autism.* Washington, DC: Author.

New York State Department of Health. (2014). *New York state early intervention program individualized family service plan.* Albany, NY: Author. Retrieved from http://cma.com/wp-content/uploads/2014/08/NYEISSampleIFSP.pdf

Newborg, J., Stock, J.R., Wnek, J., Guidubaldi, J., & Svinicki, J.S. (2002). *Battelle Developmental Inventory, Second Edition (BDI–2).* Rolling Meadows, IL: Riverside Publishing.

No Child Left Behind Act of 2001, PL 107-110, 115 Stat. 1425, 20 U.S.C. §§ 6301 *et seq.*

Norbury, C. (2014). Practitioner review: Social (pragmatic) communication disorder conceptualization, evidence and clinical implications. *Journal of Child Psychology and Psychiatry, 55,* 204–216.

Odom, S., Boyd, B., Hall, L., & Hume, K. (2010). Evaluation of comprehensive treatment models for individuals with autism spectrum disorders. *Journal of Autism and Developmental Disorders, 40,* 425–436.

Odom, S., Collet-Klinterberg, L., Rogers, S., & Hatton, D. (2010). Evidence-based practices in interventions for children and youth with autism spectrum disorders. *Preventing School Failure: Alternative Education for Children and Youth, 5*(54), 275–282.

O'Neill, R.E., Horner, R.H., Albin, R.W., Sprague, J.R., Storey, K., & Newton, J.S. (1997). *Functional assessment and program development for problem behavior: A practical handbook (2nd ed.).* Pacific Grove, CA: Brooks/Cole.

Osterling, J., & Dawson, G. (1994). Early recognition of children with autism: A study of first birthday home videotapes. *Journal of Autism and Developmental Disorders, 24,* 247–257.

Ozonoff, S., & Cathcart, K. (1998). Effectiveness of a home program intervention for young children with autism. *Journal of Autism and Developmental Disorders, 28,* 25–32.

Ozonoff, S., Heung, K., Byrd, R., Hansen, R., & Hertz-Picciotto, I. (2008). The onset of autism: Patterns of symptom emergence in the first years of life. *Autism Research, 1,* 320–328.

Ozonoff, S., Iosif, S., Baguio, F., Cook, I.C., Hill, M.H., Hutman, T. . . . Desmond, J. (2010). Preference for geometric patterns early in life as a risk factor for ASD. *Archives of General Psychiatry, 10,* 131–138.

Partington, J.W., & Sundberg, M. L. (1998). *Assessment of basic language and learning skills (The ABLLS): Instruction and IEP guide.* Pleasant Hill, CA: Behavior Analysts, Inc.

Partington, J.W., & Sundberg, M.L. (1998). *Teaching language to children with autism and other developmental disabilities.* Danville, CA: Behavior Analyst.

Patient Protection and Affordable Healthcare Act of 2010, P.L. 11-148. H.R. 3590.

Paul, R. (2009). Parents ask: Am I risking autism if I vaccinate my children? *Journal of Autism and Developmental Disorders, 39*(6), 962–963. doi: 10.1007/s10803-009-0739-y

Paul, R., Campbell, D., Tsiouri, I., & Gilbert, K. (2013). Comparing spoken language treatments for minimally verbal preschoolers with autism spectrum disorders. *Journal of Autism and Developmental Disorders, 43,* 418–431.

Paul, R., Chawarska, K., Fowler, C., Cicchetti, D., & Volkmar, F. (2007). "Listen my children and you shall hear": Auditory preferences in toddlers with autism spectrum disorders. *Journal of Speech, Language, and Hearing Research, 50*(5), 1350–1364. doi:10.1044/1092-4388(2007/094)

Paul, R. & Norbury, C. (2012). *Language disorders from infancy through adolescence: Reading, writing, listening, speaking, and communicating* (4th ed.). St. Louis: Elsevier

Pavlov, I. (2003) *Conditioned reflexes.* Translated by G.V. Anrep. Cambridge, MA: Courier Corporation.

Pickett E., Pulara, O., O'Grady, J., & Barry, G. (2009). Speech acquisition in older nonverbal individuals with autism: A review of features, methods, and prognosis. *Cognitive and Behavioral Neurology, 22,* 1–21.

Pierce, K, Conant, D, Hazin, R, Stoner, R, Desmond, J. Preference for geometric patterns early in life as a risk factor for autism. *Arch Gen Psychiatry.* 2011;68:101–109.

Prelock, P., Paul, R., & Allen, E. (2011). Evidence-based treatments in communication for children with autism spectrum disorders. In F. Volkmar & B. Reichow (Eds.), *Evidence-based treatments for children with ASD* (pp. 93–170). New York, NY: Springer.

Prizant, B., & Wetherby, A. (1989). Enhancing communication: From theory to practice. In G. Dawson (Ed.). *Autism: New perspectives on diagnosis, nature and treatment.* New York: Guilford Press.

Prizant, B.M., Wetherby, A.M., Rubin, E., Laurent, A.C., & Rydell, P.J. (2006). *The SCERTS® Model: A comprehensive educational approach for children with autism spectrum disorders.* Baltimore, MD: Paul H. Brookes Publishing Co.

Reichow, B., Barton, E.E., Neely Sewell, J., Good, L., & Wolery, M. (2010). Effects of weighted vests on the engagement of children with developmental delays and autism. *Focus on Autism and Other Developmental Disabilities, 25*(1), 3–11.

Rescorla, L. (1989). Language Development Survey (LDS). *Journal of Speech and Hearing Disorders, 54,* 587–599.

Resnick, S., Baranek, G., Reavis, S. Watson, L. & Crais, E. (2007). A parent-report instrument for identifying one-year-olds at risk for an eventual diagnosis of autism: the first year inventory. *Journal of Autism and Developmental Disorders, 37,* 1691–1710.

Robey, R. (2004). A five-phase model for clinical-outcome research. *Journal of Communication Disorders, 37,* 401–411.

Robins, D., & Dumont-Mathieu, T. (2006). Early screening for ASD: Update on the M-CHAT for autism in toddlers and other measures. *Journal of Developmental and Behavioral Pediatrics, 27,* S111–S119.

Rogers, S.J., & Dawson, G. (2009). *Play and engagement in early autism: The Early Start Denver model: Volume II: The curriculum.* New York, NY: Guilford Press.

Rogers, S., & Dawson, G. (2010). *Early Start Denver model for young children with ASD.* New York, NY: Guilford Press.

Rogers, S., Dawson, G., & Vismara, L. (2012). *An early start for your child with autism: Using everyday activities to help kids connect, communicate, and learn.* New York, NY: Guilford Press.

Rogers, S.J., Hayden, D., Hepburn, S., Charlifue-Smith, R., Hall, T., & Hayes, A. (2006). Teaching young nonverbal children with autism useful speech: A pilot study of the Denver model and PROMPT interventions. *Journal of Autism and Developmental Disorders, 36,* 1007–1024.

Rogers, S.J., & Ozonoff, S. (2014). Brief report: Symptom onset patterns and functional outcomes in young children with autism spectrum disorders. *Journal of Autism and Developmental Disorders, 41*(12), 727–1732.

Rogers, S.J., Rozga, A., Sangha, S., Sigman, M., Steinfeld, M.B., & Young, G.S. (2010). A prospective study of the emergence of early behavioral signs of autism. *Journal of the American Academy of Child and Adolescent Psychiatry, 49*(3), 256–266.

Rossetti, L. (1990). *Rossetti Infant and Toddler Language Scale.* East Moline, IL: LinguiSystems.

Rozga, A., Gutman, T., Young G., Rogers, S., Ozonoff, S., Dapretto, M., & Sigman, M. (2011). Behavioral profiles of affected and unaffected siblings of children with autism: Contribution of measures of mother-infant interaction and nonverbal communication. *Journal of Autism and Developmental Disorders, 41,* 287–301.

Rutter, M., Bailey, A., & Lord, C. (2003). *Social Communication Questionnaire (SCQ)*. Los Angeles, CA: Western Psychological Services.

Rutter, M., LeConteur, A., & Lord, C. (2003). *Autism Diagnostic Interview–Revised*. Los Angeles, CA: Western Psychological Services.

Schertz, H., & Odom, S. (2007). Promoting joint attention in toddlers with autism: A parent-mediated developmental model. *Journal of Autism and Developmental Disorders, 37,* 1562–1575.

Schopler, E., Reichler, R., & Renner, B. (1988). *Childhood Autism Rating Scale (CARS)*. Los Angeles, CA: Western Psychological Services.

Sheinkopf, S.J., & Siegel, B. (1998). Home-based behavioral treatment of young children with autism. *Journal of Autism and Developmental Disorders, 28,* 15–23.

Shore, S.M., & Grandin, T. (2003). Beyond the wall: Personal experiences with autism and Asperger syndrome (2nd ed.). Shawnee Mission, KS: Autism Asperger Publishing Company.

Shumway, S., Thurm, A., Swedo, S.E., Deprey, L., Barnett, L.A., Amaral, D.G. . . . Ozonoff, S. (2011). Brief report: Symptom onset patterns and functional outcomes in young children with autism spectrum disorders. *Journal of Autism and Developmental Disorders, 41*(12), 1727–1732.

Siegel, B. (2004). *Pervasive Developmental Disorders Screening Test–II*. San Antonio, TX: Pearson Assessments.

Siegel, B. (2007). *Helping children with autism learn: Treatment approaches for parents and professionals.* Oxford, UK: Oxford University Press.

Siller, M., Hutman, T., & Sigman, M. (2013). A parent-mediated intervention to increase responsive parental behaviors and child communication in children with ASD: A randomized clinical trial. *Journal of Autism and Developmental Disorders, 43*(3), 540–555.

Skinner, B.F. (1965). *Science and human behavior.* New York, NY: Free Press Publishing.

Solish, A., Perry, A., & Minnes, P. (2010). Participation of children with and without disabilities in social recreational, and leisure activities. *Journal of Applied Research in Intellectual Disabilities, 23,* 226–126

Solomon, R., Necheles, J., Ferch, C., & Bruckman, D. (2007). Pilot study of a parent training program for young children with autism. *Autism, 11,* 205–224.

Stephenson, J., Carter, M. (2009). The use of weighted vests with children with autism spectrum disorders and other disabilities. *Journal of Autism and Developmental Disorders, 39,* 105–114.

Stone, W., Conrood, E., Pozdol, S., & Turner, L. (2004). The Parent Interview for Autism-Clinical Version (PIA-CV): A Measure of Behavioral Change for Young Children with Autism. *Journal of Autism and Developmental Disorders, 6,* 691–701.

Strain, P., & Bovey, E. (2011). Randomized, controlled trial of the LEAP model of early intervention with young children with ASD. *Topics in Early Childhood Special Education, 31,* 133–154.

Sundberg, M. L. (2008) *Verbal behavior milestones assessment and placement program: The VB-MAPP.* Concord, CA: AVB Press.

Suskind, R. (2014). *Life, animated: A story of sidekicks, heroes, and autism.* New York, NY: Kingswell Publishers.

Tammet, D., *Born on a blue day.* (2007). New York, NY: Free Press Publishing.

Taylor, J.L., & Seltzer, M.M. (2011). Employment and post-secondary educational activities for young adults with autism spectrum disorders during the transition to adulthood. *Journal of Autism and Developmental Disorders, 41*(5), 566–574. doi:10.1007/s10803-010-1070-3

The Developmental Disabilities Assistance and Bill of Rights Act of 2000. P.L. 106-492. 114 Stat. 1677

Tsiouri, I.G., & Paul, R. (2012). *Rapid Motor Imitation Antecedent (RMIA) training manual, research edition: Teaching preverbal children with ASD to talk.* Baltimore, MD: Paul H. Brookes Publishing Co.

Uddin, L.Q., Supekar, K., & Menon, V. (2013). Reconceptualizing functional brain connectivity in autism from a developmental perspective. *Frontiers in Human Neuroscience, 7.* doi:10.3389/fnhum.2013.00458

Unumb, L., & Unumb, D. (2011). *Autism and the law: Cases, statutes, and materials.* Durham, NC: Carolina Academic Press.

U.S. Department of Defense Education Activity. (2005). DoDEA Form 2500.13-G-F26: Individualized education program (IEP). Alexandria, VA: Author. Retrieved from http://www.dodea.edu/Curriculum/specialEduc/upload/DoDEAForm2500-13-G-F26.pdf

Volkmar, F., Reichow, B., Westphal, A., & Mandell, D. (2013). Autism and the autism spectrum: Diagnostic concepts. In F. Volkmar, S. Rogers, R. Paul, & K. Pelphrey (Eds.), *Handbook of autism and pervasive developmental disorders* (4th ed.; pp. 3–27). New York, NY: Wiley.

Volkmar, F., & Weisner, L. (2009). *A practical guide to autism: What every parent, family member, and teacher needs to know.* New York, NY: Wiley.

Wagner, A., Wallace, K., & Rogers, S. (2014). Developmental approaches to treatment of young children with autism spectrum disorder. In J. Tarbox, D. Dixon, P. Sturmey, & J. Matson (Eds.), *Handbook of early intervention for autism spectrum disorders: Autism and child psychopathology series* (pp. 393–427). New York, NY: Springer.

Warren, S., Bredin-Oja, S., Fairchild, M., Finestack, L., Fey, M., and Brady, N. (2006). Responsivity education/prelinguistic milieu teaching. In R. McCauley and M. Fey (Eds.). *Treatment of language disorders in children* (pp. 47–75). Baltimore, MD: Paul H. Brookes Publishing Co.

Watson, J. (1913). Psychology as the behaviorist views it. *Psychological Review, 20,* 158–177.

Wetherby, A. (2009). *Video glossary.* http://www.autismspeaks.org/what-autism/video-glossary

Wetherby, A. & Prizant, B. (2002). *Communication and Symbolic Behavior Scales Developmental Profile™ (CSBS DP™).* Baltimore, MD: Paul H. Brookes Publishing Co.

Wetherby, A., Prizant, B., & Hutchinson, T. (1998). Communicative, social/affective, and symbolic profiles of young children with autism and pervasive developmental disorders. *American Journal of Speech-Language Pathology, 7,* 79–91.

Wetherby, A.M., & Woods, J. (2006). Early social interaction project for children with autism spectrum disorders beginning in the second year of life: A preliminary study. *Topics in Early Childhood Special Education, 26,* 67–82.

Wishman, N. (2009). *Red flags.* http://www.firstsigns.org/concerns/flags.htm

Wolf, S. (2004). The history of autism. *European Child and Adolescent Psychiatry, 13,* 201–208.

Wong, C., Odom. S., Hume, K., Cox, C., Fettig, A., Kurchararczyk, S., Brock, M., Plavnick, F., Fleury, V., & Schultz, T. (2015). Evidence-based practices for children, youth, and young adults with autism spectrum disorders: A comprehensive review. *Journal of Autism and Developmental Disorders,* Advance online publication. doi: 10.1007/s10803-014-2351-z.

Wright, P.W.D., & Wright, D. (2007). *Winkelman v. Parma City School Dist. (6th Cir. 2006).* Retrieved from http://www.wrightslaw.com/law/caselaw/06/6th.winkelman.parma.oh.htm.

Yoder, P., & Stone, W. (2006). Randomized comparison of two communication interventions for preschoolers with autism spectrum disorders. *Journal of Consulting and Clinical Psychology, 74,* 426–435.

Zimmerman, I., Steiner, V., & Pond, R. (2011). *Preschool Language Scale—Fifth Edition (PLS-5).* San Antonio, TX: Pearson/Harcourt Assessment.

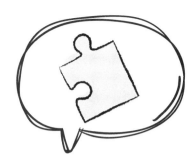

Suggested Resources

RESOURCES FOR FAMILIES OF CHILDREN WITH ASD (CHAPTER 1)

Autism Consortium	http://www.autismconsortium.org/families/family-supports
Autism Diario (for English- and Spanish-speaking families)	http://autismodiario.org
Autism Friendly Spaces	http://autismfriendlyspaces.org
Autism Now	http://autismnow.org/at-home/family/support-at-home
Autism Society of America	http://www.autism-society.org
Autism Speaks	http://www.autismspeaks.org/family-services/tool-kits/family-support-tool-kits
First Signs	http://www.firstsigns.org
Interactive Autism Network	http://www.iancommunity.org
Jewish Autism Trust	http://www.jewishautism.org
New York Families for Autistic Children	http://nyfac.org
Organization for Autism Research	http://www.researchautism.org/family/familysupport/index.asp
We Care	http://www.wecarechildren.org/contact

RESOURCES FOR EDUCATIONAL PLANNING (CHAPTER 5)

Interagency Council of Developmental Disabilities Agencies	http://www.iacny.org
Social Security	http://www.ssa.gov/planners/ benefitcalculators.htm
Social Security: Benefits for Children with Disabilities	http://www.ssa.gov/pubs/EN-05 -10026.pdf
The ARC of the United States	http://www.thearc.org/page.aspx?pid =3044
U.S. Department of Education, Office of Special Education and Rehabilitative Services	http://www2.ed.gov/about/offices/list/ osers/osep/index.html?src=mr
ZERO TO THREE, National Center for Infants, Toddlers, and Families	http://www.zerotothree.org
The Developmental Disabilities Assistance and Bill of Rights Act of 2000	http://www.acl.gov/Programs/AIDD/ DDA_BOR_ACT_2000/Index .aspx

RESOURCES FOR FAMILIES ON TREATMENT RESEARCH (CHAPTER 7)

Association for Science in Autism Treatment	http://www.asatonline.org
Autism Intervention Research Network on Physical Health	http://www.airpnetwork.org/site/ c.70JGLPPsFiJYG/b.8238437/k .BEBF/Home.htm?sid=366854572
Autism Speaks	http://www.autismspeaks.org
Autism Watch	http://www.autism-watch.org
National Research Council Report	http://www.nap.edu/openbook.php ?isbn=0309072697
Recommendations of Expert Panels and Government Task Force	http://www.asatonline.org/for -parents/learn-more-about -specific-treatments/applied -behavior-analysis-aba/ aba-techniques/recommendations -of-expert-panels-government -task-forces/

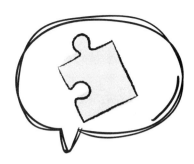

Index

Tables and figures are indicated by *t* and *f*, respectively.